Anatomy & Physiology

2,000
Quiz & Puzzle Questions
For Exam Success

By

Kate L Tierney

© Anatomy & Physiology Student Workbook 2013

The right of Kate L. Tierney to be identified as author of his work has been asserted by him in accordance with the Copyright, Designs and Patents Act 1988.

All rights reserved; no part of this publication may be reproduced, stored in a retrieval system, or transmitted in any form or by any means, electronic, mechanical, photocopying, recording or otherwise without the prior written permission of the publisher.

First published in Octobor 2007
Revised Edition: February 2013

ISBN-13: 978-1468175806
ISBN-10: 1468175807

Contents

1. The Cell - Pg 6
2. The Skin - Pg 32
3. The Skeletal System - Pg 60
4. The Muscular System - Pg 85
5. The Cardiovascular System - Pg 120
6. The Lymphatic System - Pg 141
7. The Endocrine System - Pg 156
8. The Nervous System - Pg 178
9. The Reproductive System - Pg 197
10. The Respiratory System - Pg 217
11. The Digestive System - Pg 236
12. The Urinary System - Pg 256
13. Mock Exam Papers - Pg 271

Introduction

This book is aimed at students studying towards Holistic or Beauty Qualifications. It has been designed as a revision resource, which should be used in conjunction with class text books.

There are 13 chapters, with a total of 1,160 Multiple Choice Questions. Each question has 4 possible answers, with an answer grid at the end of each chapter. You will also be able to practice for your exams by completing the 58 crosswords provided. With hundreds of clues covering all systems of the body, these puzzles are designed to be repeated several times until your confidence grows.

Anatomy & Physiology, 1,160 MCQ is considered to be one of the most popular and successful anatomy & physiology revision guides on the market today, having already assisted thousands of students worldwide in completing their exams with ease.

Test yourself daily with a mixture of questions. Do this regularly and you will find the subject of anatomy & physiology becoming a little easier to manage.

Other Books in the Series

Anatomy & Physiology Workbook - 1,160 Multiple Choice Questions, by Kate L. Tierney

Anatomy & Physiology Essential Revision - 4,000 Revision Questions, Level 4 - Level 5, co-written by Gerard T. Lucas & Kate L. Tierney

Anatomy & Physiology Essential Revision Study Companion - 1,000 Glossary of Terms, co-written by Gerard T. Lucas & Kate L. Tierney (available on Kindle only).

Chapter 1 | The Cell & Tissues

Revision Puzzles & Questions

Exercise 1

The following grid lists statements on the left that are either true or false. Please choose your answer on the right. All answers are provided at the end of the chapter.

1.	A group of cells join to form an organ	True ☐ False ■
2.	Anaphase is the second stage of mitosis	True ☐ False ■
3.	Mitochondria supply the cell with its energy	True ■ False ☐
4.	Support and secretion are important functions of a cell	True ☐ False ■
5.	Lymphoid tissue is a type of connective tissue	True ■ False ☐
6.	Osmosis describes the movement of water through the cell membrane from an area of high concentration until the concentration is equal on both sides	True ■ False ☐
7.	Cell multiplication is known as mitosis	True ■ False ☐

Anatomy & Physiology Student Workbook

8.	Columnar epithelium are cells which line the respiratory system	True ☐ False ☒
9.	Ribosomes produce proteins to use within the cell	True ☒ False ☐
10.	After fertilisation the sperm and the egg fuse together to form an embryo	True ☐ False ☒
11.	The cell divides into 2 cells in the metaphase of mitosis	True ☐ False ☒
12.	Ribosomes destroy harmful bacteria and worn out parts of the cell	True ☐ False ☒
13.	The nucleus is known as the control centre of the cell	True ☒ False ☐
14.	Adipose and areolar tissue are types of connective tissue	True ☒ False ☐
15.	ATP is formed within the mitochondria and is responsible for the production of protein	True ☐ False ☒
16.	Simple epithelium consists of a single layer of thin, flattened cells attached to a basement membrane	True ☒ False ☐
17.	Chromosomes are formed during the anaphase	True ☒ False ☐

Anatomy & Physiology Student Workbook

18.	A group of tissues join to form a system	True ☐ False ☒
19.	A zygote has 23 chromosomes	True ☐ False ☒
20.	Fibrous tissue is found in the lining of the heart	True ☐ False ☒
21.	Yellow elastic cartilage is found in areas where flexibility is needed	True ☒ False ☐
22.	Sex cell division is known as meiosis	True ☐ False ☐
23.	Non keratinised stratified epithelium is found on dry surfaces, e.g. nails	True ☐ False ☐
24.	Diffusion occurs when small molecules pass through tiny pores in the cell membrane	True ☐ False ☐
25.	The cytoplasm controls what substances are passed out of the cell such as carbon dioxide	True ☐ False ☐
26.	Ciliated epithelium have fine, hair like projections called cilia attached to its surface	True ☐ False ☐
27.	Smooth ER and rough ER are types of endoplasmic reticulum	True ☐ False ☐

28.	The cell is the basic unit of life	True ☐ False ☐
29.	Ribosomes are empty spaces within the cytoplasm	True ☐ False ☐
30.	Squamous epithelium lines the alveoli of the lungs	True ☐ False ☐
31.	The cytoplasm surrounds the cell membrane supplying it with nutrients for growth and repair	True ☐ False ☐
32.	Simple and compound are 2 types of epithelial tissue	True ☐ False ☐
33.	Yellow elastic cartilage forms the intervertebral discs of the spine	True ☐ False ☐
34.	Centrioles play an important part in cell division and are contained within the golgi apparatus	True ☐ False ☐
35.	Adipose tissue helps to form tendons which attach muscle to bone	True ☐ False ☐
36.	Filtration occurs when there is a difference in pressure on each side of the membrane, causing the movement of water and dissolved substances across the membrane	True ☐ False ☐

37.	Telophase is the third phase of mitosis	True ☐ False ☐
38.	Columnar epithelium is found in the kidney tubules, ovaries, thyroid gland and salivary glands	True ☐ False ☐
39.	Histology describes the study of cells and tissues	True ☐ False ☐
40.	The term catabolism refers to the chemical breakdown of large, complex substances into smaller, simpler ones	True ☐ False ☐

Exercise 2

Match the types of tissues, cells and cartilage with each of their functions. Please choose your answers from the box at the end of this exercise.

1.	Cells which help to move unwanted particles away from the lungs, keeping passageways clear	
2.	Tissue which is protective, provides insulation and is an energy reserve	
3.	A type of cartilage that contains chondrocytes and is found on the surfaces of the end of bones that form joints	
4.	The most solid of all connective tissues, it supports and protects the body	
5.	Epithelium which provides lubrication	
6.	Tissue which helps to protect the body from infection	
7.	Cells involved in the secretion and absorption of mucus	
8.	A type of epithelium whose cells can change shape when they are stretched	
9.	A strong tissue made up of collagen fibres that forms tendons and ligaments and provides a protective outer covering for organs	
10.	A flexible cartilage, which maintains its shape	

Anatomy & Physiology Student Workbook

11.	A type of epithelium with flattened cells that line the alveoli of the lungs	Squamous
12.	A type of connective tissue that is found in most parts of the body	Areolar
13.	A type of tissue that contains neurones and is responsible for co-ordinating and controlling the body's activities	Nervous
14.	Stratified epithelium that protects the underlying tissues and prevents them from drying out	Keratinised Stratified
15.	Tissue where elasticity is required to enable the stretching of various organs	Transitional
16.	A liquid connective tissue that transports nutrients throughout the body, fights infection and forms clots	Blood
17.	A type of simple epithelium that is responsible for the absorption and secretion of substances	Columnar
18.	Tissue which maintains posture and moves the body	Muscle
19.	Cartilage that forms the intervertebral discs	White Fibrocartilage

Please choose your answers from this grid

Blood	Areolar	White Fibrous Cartilage	Muscle
Cuboidal	Squamous	Non Keratinised Stratified	White Fibrous
Adipose	Transitional	Hyaline	Yellow Elastic
Ciliated	Nervous	Keratinised Stratified	Bone
Lymphoid	Columnar	Yellow Elastic Fibrocartilage	

Exercise 3

Complete the following crossword on The Cell by answering the clues below.

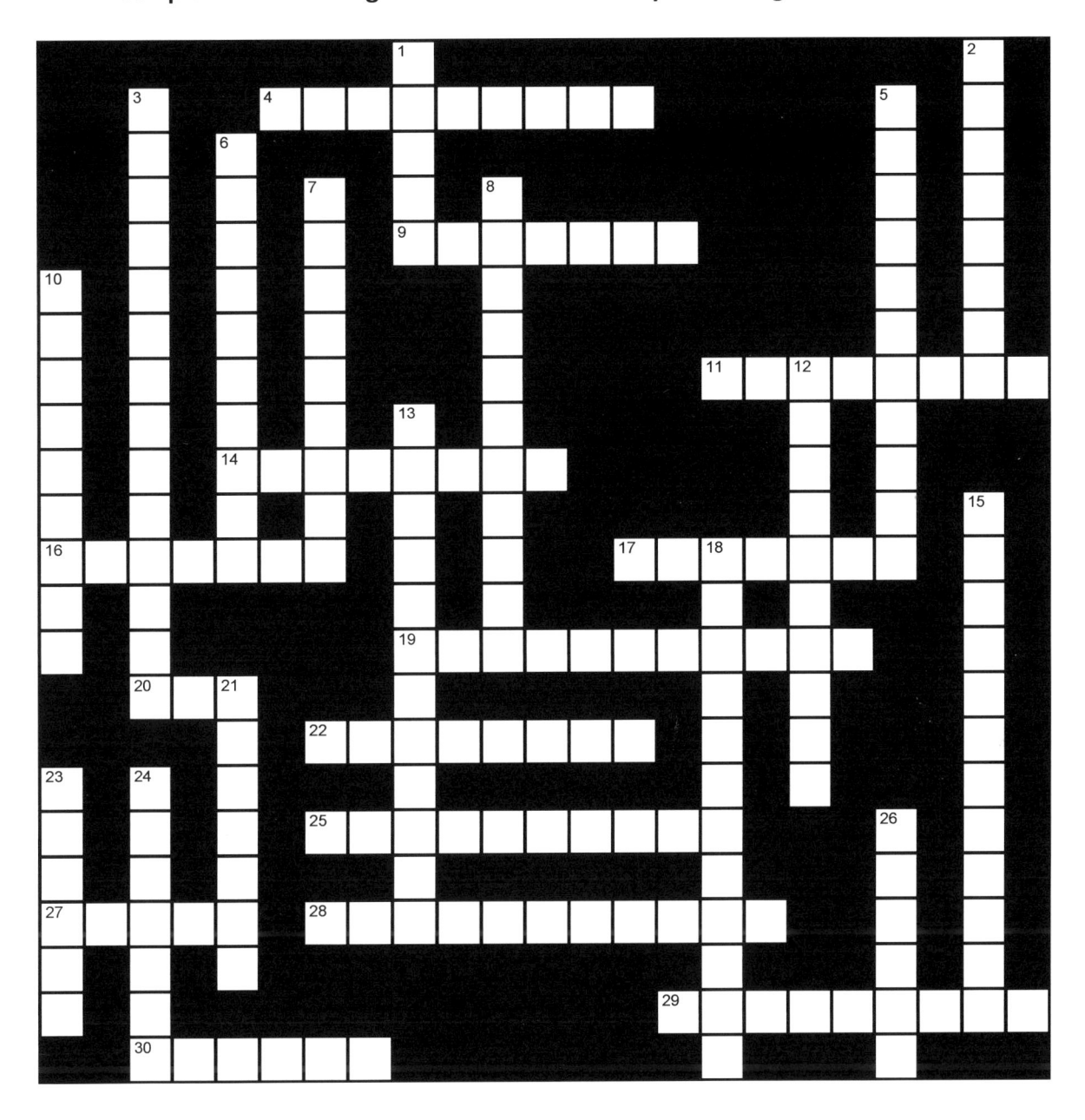

Across
4. What substance contains the nucleus and organelles? (9)
9. What type of cartilage is found on the end of bones where joints are formed? (7)
11. Empty sacs within the cytoplasm (8)
14. What type of connective tissue contains lymphocytes? (8)
16. A type of cell division involved with sexual reproduction (7)
17. What part of the cell is responsible for control of the cell's growth and repair? (7)
19. What is the function of white fibrocartilage? (11)

20. What do chromosomes contain? (3)
22. What type of simple epithelium can absorb and secrete substances? (8)
25. What is the living content inside a cell called? (10)
27. The smallest units of matter (5)
28. What system of the body is lined with ciliated cells? (11)
29. The creation of complex molecules from simpler ones (9)
30. What phase of mitosis is the metaphase? (6)

Down
1. There are 2 types of endoplasmic reticulum, which one has ribosomes present? (5)
2. What phase of mitosis do sets of chromosomes assemble to each pole of the cell? (8)
3. What type of stratified epithelium can be found in the lining of the mouth? (14)
5. What are the mitochondria known as? (11)
6. Cylindrical cell structures that sit on opposite sides of the nucleus (10)
7. Organelles that contain digestive enzymes and break down waste for elimination (9)
8. Another term for adipose tissue (11)
10. What part of the cell manufactures proteins? (9)
12. What is the most common type of tissue found in the body that has important protection and support functions? (10)
13. What type of connective tissue is made up of collagen fibres? (12)
15. What types of cells are found in hyaline cartilage? (12)
18. What substance protects the cell's contents and oversees the exchange of nutrients and waste in and out of the cell? (12)
21. What type of tissue helps to protect the loss of body heat? (7)
23. What do a group of tissues joined together form? (6)
24. The movement of substances through the cell membrane from an area of low concentration to high concentration until both sides are equal (7)
26. What type of epithelium do ciliated and columnar fall under? (6)

Exercise 4

Match the types of tissues and cartilage with the locations of where they are found on the body. Please choose your answers from the box at the end of this exercise.

1.	Under the skin and in the alimentary canal	
2.	Intervertebral discs	
3.	Lymph nodes, spleen and tonsils	
4.	At the ends of long bones that form joints	
5.	Inside the mouth and conjunctiva of the eyes	
6.	Lining of the heart and blood vessels	
7.	Bladder and uterus	
8.	The respiratory system	
9.	Ligaments	
10.	Stomach and small intestine	
11.	Hair, nails and skin	
12.	Pinna and epiglottis	

| 13. | Kidney tubules and ovaries | |

Please choose your answers from this grid

Areolar	Cuboidal	Ciliated	Yellow Elastic
White Fibrous	Lymphoid	Transitional	Keratinised
Squamous	Non Keratinised	Columnar	Hyaline
White Fibrocartilage			

Exercise 5

Please answer the questions below and find the answers in the word search puzzle.

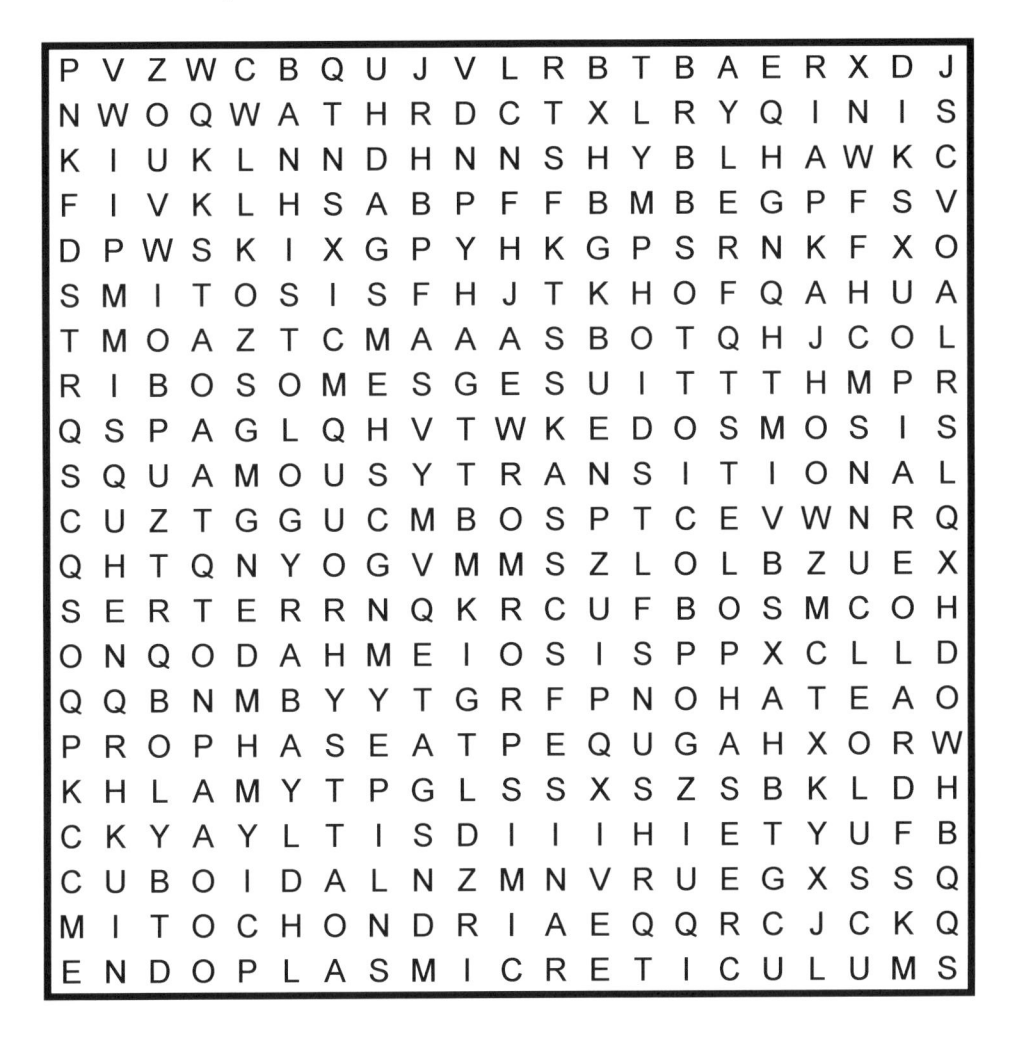

```
P V Z W C B Q U J V L R B T B A E R X D J
N W O Q W A T H R D C T X L R Y Q I N I S
K I U K L N N D H N N S H Y B L H A W K C
F I V K L H S A B P F F B M B E G P F S V
D P W S K I X G P Y H K G P S R N K F X O
S M I T O S I S F H J T K H O F Q A H U A
T M O A Z T C M A A A S B O T Q H J C O L
R I B O S O M E S G E S U I T T T H M P R
Q S P A G L Q H V T W K E D O S M O S I S
S Q U A M O U S Y T R A N S I T I O N A L
C U Z T G G U C M B O S P T C E V W N R Q
Q H T Q N Y O G V M M S Z L O L B Z U E X
S E R T E R R N Q K R C U F B O S M C O H
O N Q O D A H M E I O S I S P P X C L L D
Q Q B N M B Y Y T G R F P N O H A T E A O
P R O P H A S E A T P E Q U G A H X O R W
K H L A M Y T P G L S S X S Z S B K L D H
C K Y A Y L T I S D I I I H I E T Y U F B
C U B O I D A L N Z M N V R U E G X S S Q
M I T O C H O N D R I A E Q Q R C J C K Q
E N D O P L A S M I C R E T I C U L U M S
```

1. What is the study of the anatomy of cells and tissues? (9)
2. What describes the process of transferring substances from a low to high concentration until they are equal on each side? (7)
3. What organelles produce the cell's power? (12)
4. What are the protein synthesizers of a cell? (9)
5. What part of the cell is responsible for the transport of cellular materials? (20)
6. What structure forms ribosomes? (9)
7. A substance found in the nucleus of a cell, composed of DNA and proteins (9)
8. What do grouped together tissues form? (5)
9. What is the term used to describe cell reproduction? (7)
10. What is the third phase of mitosis? (8)
11. During what stage of mitosis does the nuclear membrane start to break down? (8)
12. What type of connective tissue helps to protect against disease? (8)
13. What type of compound epithelium is found in organs that need to change shape? (12)

14. What types of cells are found within hyaline cartilage? (12)
15. What is the most widely distributed connective tissue found in the body? (7)
16. What type of simple epithelium contains a single layer of flattened cells? (8)
17. At what stage of mitosis do the spindle fibres disappear? (9)
18. What is the reproduction of sex cells called? (7)
19. What type of simple epithelium lines the kidney tubules? (8)
20. What type of cartilage is found on the ends of bones that form joints? (7)

Exercise 6

Please fill in the missing words:

1. During the metaphase of mitosis the _____ _____ disappears completely (7,8)

2. The stomach and intestines are lined with _____ epithelium (8)

3. ATP is the main provider of _____ within the cell (6)

4. The _____ _____ stores the protein received from the endoplasmic reticulum and later transports it out of the cell (5,9)

5. The telophase is the _____ of mitosis (6)

6. During the _____ of mitosis the chromatids are stretched further apart, moving to each end of the cell (8)

7. _____ _____ tissue enables organs to be stretched and returned to their original shape (6,7)

8. A group of cells join together to form _____ (6)

9. Human cells contain _____ chromosomes (2)

10. During the prophase of mitosis pairs of _____ become visible (11)

11. Fatty tissue is also known as _____ tissue (7)

12. Ciliated epithelium lines the _____ system (11)

13. Vacuoles contain _____ spaces within the cytoplasm (5)

14. The _____ is known as the brain of the cell, controlling the cell's activities (7)

15. The _____ is the first phase of mitosis (8)

Exercise 7

Please answer the questions in the grid by matching the answers in the box at the end of this exercise.

1.	During which stage of mitosis do the chromosomes align themselves in the middle of the cell, each attached to the spindle fibre by its centromere?	
2.	What type of epithelium has one layer of cells connected to a basement membrane?	
3.	What type of tissue forms tendons and ligaments?	
4.	What part of the cell digests all parts of the cell that are old and worn out?	
5.	What do a group of organs join to form?	
6.	What is the second phase of mitosis?	
7.	What type of connective tissue provides heat protection and acts as an energy reserve?	
8.	What type of stratified epithelium provides lubrication?	
9.	What part of the cell is used for storage?	

10.	What do a group of systems join together to form?	
11.	During what stage of mitosis does a new nuclear envelope form around each set of chromosomes?	
12.	What type of simple epithelium lines the heart?	
13.	What tissue of the body provides support and protection?	
14.	Pairs of microtubules that sit at right angles next to each other, moving towards the opposite ends of the nucleus during mitosis	
15.	What type of stratified epithelium prevents underlying layers of cells from drying out before they reach the surface of the skin?	

Please choose your answers from this grid

Adipose	Metaphase	System
Simple	Lysosomes	Telophase
Organism	Connective	Vacuoles
Centrioles	White Fibrous	Metaphase
Non Keratinised	Squamous	Keratinised

Exercise 8

Multiple choice questions, please choose one answer from the 4 choices provided in each box.

1. What type of endoplasmic reticulum manufactures steroids and lipids? a) Smooth b) Columnar c) Ciliated d) Rough Answer: ~~C~~ A	**2. What part of the cell contains enzymes which destroy bacteria and wastes?** a) Chromatin b) Mitochondria c) Lysosomes d) Vacuoles Answer: ~~b~~ C
3. Which one of the following is a function of a cell? a) Growth b) Maintain posture c) Secretion d) Absorption Answer: a	**4. A group of tissues join to form;** a) Cell b) Organ c) System d) Nucleus Answer: b
5. Squamous epithelium; a) Are cube shaped cells b) Are tall, cylindrical shaped cells c) Are flat, thin cells d) Are columnar shaped cells Answer: ~~A~~ C	**6. How is glucose transferred through the cell membrane?** a) Osmosis b) Filtration c) Dissolution d) Active transport Answer: D
7. Which one of the following is a type of connective tissue? a) Nervous b) Muscular c) Chromosomes d) Lymphoid Answer: ~~B~~ D	**8. What is the final stage of mitosis?** a) Telophase b) Anaphase c) Prophase d) Metaphase Answer: ~~C~~ A

9. Define Anabolism;	10. What supplies the cell with its energy?
a) The process by which complex substances are broken down into simpler substances	a) Vacuoles
b) The process by which larger substances which cannot pass through the cell membrane are dissolved	b) Endoplasmic reticulum
c) The process by which simpler molecules are built up into complex molecules	c) Mitochondria
d) The process by which water moves through the cell membrane from an area of high to low concentration until the concentration is equal on both sides	d) Golgi apparatus
Answer: C	Answer: A C
11. What is the control centre of the cell?	12. Which type of compound epithelium is found lining the alveoli of the lungs?
a) Cytoplasm	a) Columnar
b) Nucleus	b) Cuboidal
c) Mitochondria	c) Ciliated
d) Ribosomes	d) Squamous
Answer: B	Answer: C D
13. During which phase of mitosis are chromosomes formed?	14. What is responsible for the formation of ribosomes?
a) Metaphase	a) Nucleolus
b) Anaphase	b) Lysosomes
c) Prophase	c) Nucleus
d) Telophase	d) Chromatin
Answer: A C	Answer: B A

15. Where is all genetic information needed to make a person, stored?
a) ATP
b) DNA
c) RNA
d) EAC

Answer: B

16. What is the correct order of mitosis?
a) Metaphase, anaphase, telophase, prophase
b) Prophase, metaphase, anaphase, telophase
c) Anaphase, prophase, metaphase, telophase
d) Prophase, metaphase, telophase, anaphase

Answer: A B

17. A protein found in skin, hair and nails;
a) Yellow elastic
b) Hyaline
c) Squamous
d) Keratin

Answer: D

18. Where can yellow elastic cartilage be found in the body?
a) Hip and shoulder sockets
b) Nose and trachea
c) Pinna and epiglottis
d) Heart and kidney tubules

Answer: B C

19. What is the most general type of connective tissue found in the body?
a) Areolar
b) Lymphoid
c) Adipose
d) Yellow elastic

Answer: A

20. Simple epithelium consists of;
a) A single layer of cells
b) Several layers of cells
c) 2 layers of flattened cells
d) 2 layers of cuboidal cells

Answer: A

21. Which one of the following is not a way in which substances can pass in and out of cells?
a) Osmosis
b) Dissolution
c) Filtration
d) Mitosis

Answer: B D

22. Where would you find centrioles?
a) Within centrosomes
b) Within smooth endoplasmic reticulum
c) Within mitochondria
d) Within the chromosomes

Answer: D A

Anatomy & Physiology Student Workbook

23. A jelly like substance composed mainly of water; a) Cell membrane b) Cytoplasm c) Mitochondria d) Epithelium Answer: B	**24.** What is the most common type of cartilage? a) Yellow elastic b) White c) Hyaline d) Fibrocartilage Answer: C
25. What does the golgi apparatus store? a) Cytoplasm b) Tissue c) Protein d) DNA Answer: C	**26.** What is the function of ribosomes? a) To control the growth of the cell b) To manufacture protein c) To destroy bacteria d) To supply the cell with energy Answer: B
27. What part of the cell produces energy? a) Lysosomes b) Mitochondria c) Endoplasmic reticulum d) Nucleus Answer: B	**28.** Centrioles separate and move toward the end of the cell during what stage of mitosis? a) Prophase b) Telophase c) Anaphase d) Metaphase Answer: A
29. Which connective tissue connects skin to underlying skin and muscles? a) Lymphoid b) Bone c) White fibrous d) Areolar Answer: D	**30.** What are the empty spaces within the cytoplasm called? a) Lysosomes b) Centrioles c) Vacuoles d) Nucleolus Answer: C

31. What is the largest organelle in a cell? a) Cytoplasm b) Nucleolus c) Mitochondria d) Nucleus Answer: D C	**32. What type of cells are found in lymphoid tissue?** a) Lymphocytes b) Fibrocytes c) Mast cells d) Red blood cells Answer: D
33. What type of cartilage is flexible? a) Yellow elastic b) Hyaline c) Fibrocartilage d) Synovial Answer: A	**34. What protects the cell's contents?** a) Nucleus b) Cell membrane c) Chromatin d) Cytoplasm Answer: B
35. A fluid connective tissue; a) Areolar b) Adipose c) Bone d) Blood Answer: B D	**36. The process by which small molecules pass through the cell membrane from an area of high concentration to an area of low concentration is known as;** a) Active transport b) Filtration c) Diffusion d) Osmosis Answer: D C
37. Where can non keratinised stratified epithelium be found? a) Hair b) Bladder c) Lining of the mouth d) Nails Answer: B C	**38. How many chromosomes are in a cell before fertilisation?** a) 23 b) 46 c) 18 d) 22 Answer: A

39. Where can transitional epithelium be found?	40. Which one of the following is a function of connective tissue?
a) Heart	a) Movement
b) Bladder	b) Secretion
c) Pharynx	c) Lubrication
d) Thyroid gland	d) Protection
Answer: B	Answer: D

The Cell & Tissues

Answers

Exercise 1 (true/false):

1. False	11. False	21. True	31. False
2. False	12. False	22. True	32. True
3. True	13. True	23. False	33. False
4. False	14. True	24. True	34. False
5. True	15. False	25. False	35. False
6. True	16. True	26. True	36. True
7. True	17. True	27. True	37. False
8. False	18. False	28. True	38. False
9. True	19. False	29. False	39. True
10. False	20. False	30. True	40. True

Exercises 2 (match the types of tissues/cartilage/cells):

1. Ciliated
2. Adipose
3. Hyaline
4. Bone
5. Non Keratinised
6. Lymphoid
7. Columnar
8. Transitional
9. White Fibrous
10. Yellow Elastic
11. Squamous
12. Areolar
13. Nervous
14. Keratinised
15. Yellow Elastic
16. Blood
17. Cuboidal
18. Muscle
19. White Fibrous

Exercise 3 (Crossword):

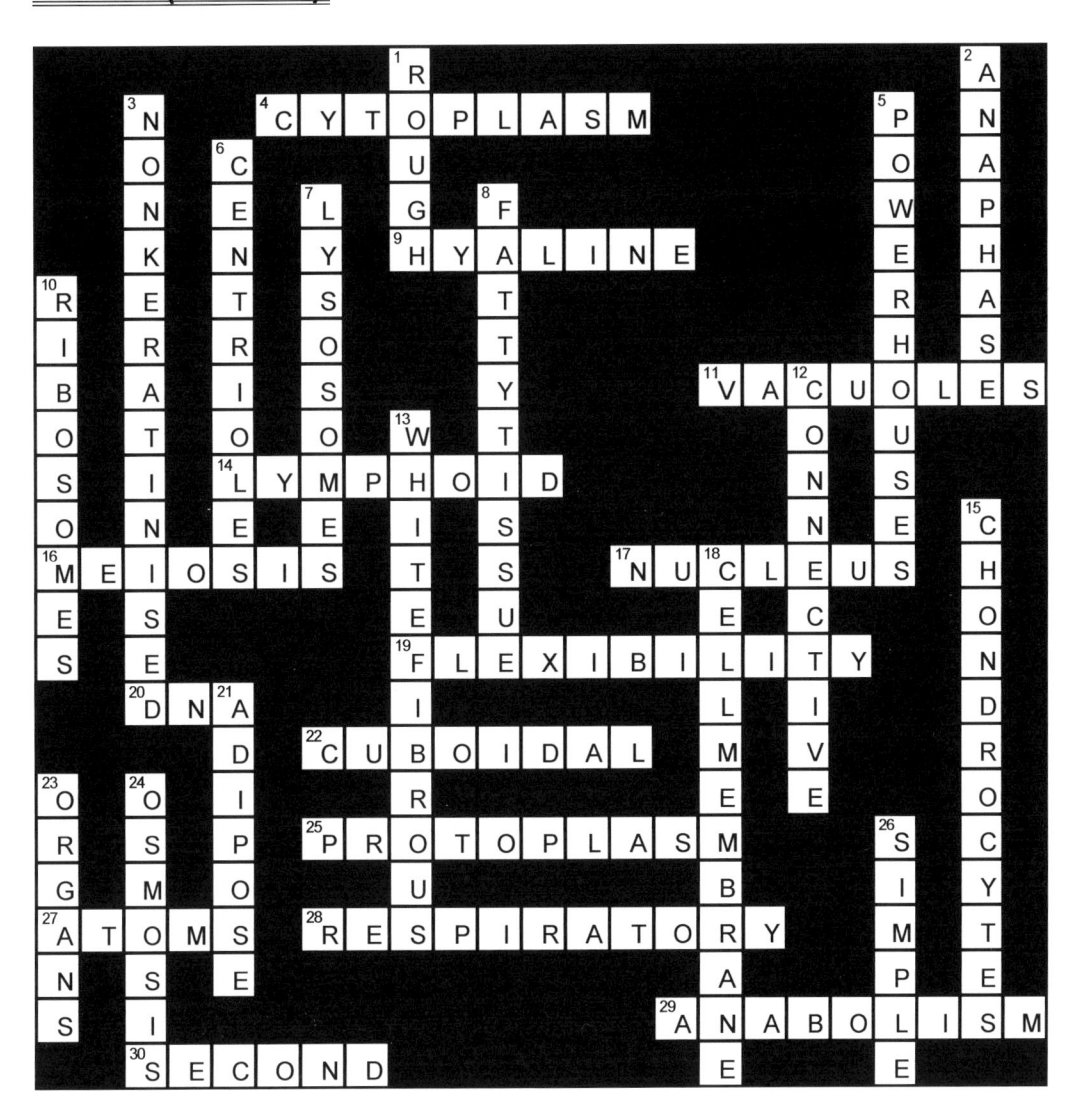

Exercise 4 (match tissues/cartilages with the locations in the body):

1. Areolar
2. White Fibrocartilage
3. Lymphoid
4. Hyaline
5. Non Keratinised
6. Squamous
7. Transitional
8. Ciliated
9. White Fibrous
10. Columnar
11. Keratinised
12. Yellow Elastic
13. Cuboidal

Exercise 5 (Word Search Puzzle):

1. Histology
2. Osmosis
3. Mitochondria
4. Ribosomes
5. Endoplasmic Reticulum
6. Nucleolus
7. Chromatin
8. Organ
9. Mitosis
10. Anaphase
11. Prophase
12. Lymphoid
13. Transitional
14. Chondrocytes
15. Areolar
16. Squamous
17. Telophase
18. Meiosis
19. Cuboidal
20. Hyaline

Exercise 6 (fill in the missing words):

1. Nuclear membrane
2. Columnar
3. Energy
4. Golgi Apparatus
5. Fourth
6. Anaphase
7. Yellow Elastic
8. Tissue
9. 46
10. Chromosomes
11. Adipose
12. Respiratory
13. Empty
14. Nucleus
15. Prophase

Exercise 7 (match answers with questions in the grid):

1. Metaphase
2. Simple
3. White Fibrous
4. Lysosomes
5. System
6. Metaphase
7. Adipose
8. Non Keratinised
9. Vacuoles
10. Organism
11. Telophase
12. Squamous
13. Connective
14. Centrioles
15. Keratinised

Exercise 8 (multiple choice questions):

1	A	9	C	17	D	25	C	33	A
2	C	10	C	18	C	26	B	34	B
3	A	11	B	19	A	27	B	35	D
4	B	12	D	20	A	28	A	36	C
5	C	13	C	21	D	29	D	37	C
6	D	14	A	22	A	30	C	38	A
7	D	15	B	23	B	31	D	39	B
8	A	16	B	24	C	32	A	40	D

Chapter 2 | Skin, Hair & Nails

Revision Puzzles & Questions

Exercise 1

The following grid lists statements on the left that are either true or false. Please choose your answer on the right. All answers are provided at the end of the chapter.

1.	The basal cell layer is known as the stratum germinativum	True ☐ False ☐
2.	Milia are commonly found on oily, greasy skin	True ☐ False ☐
3.	Impetigo is a contagious bacterial infection	True ☐ False ☐
4.	Protection is a function of the skin	True ☐ False ☐
5.	Desquamation occurs in the stratum lucidum	True ☐ False ☐
6.	Apocrine glands are located on the palms of the hands	True ☐ False ☐
7.	The skin is the largest organ in the body	True ☐ False ☐

8.	Vitiligo is a pigmentation disorder in which the skin and hair cannot produce melanin	True ☐ False ☐
9.	Melanin is produced by melanocytes in the stratum germinativum	True ☐ False ☐
10.	The temperature of the body should be constantly maintained at 36.8°C	True ☐ False ☐
11.	The reticular layer of the dermis contains collagen and elastin fibres	True ☐ False ☐
12.	Ephelides are also called blackheads	True ☐ False ☐
13.	Acne vulgaris is a viral infection	True ☐ False ☐
14.	The epidermis is the layer of the skin that we can see and touch	True ☐ False ☐
15.	It takes approximately 2 weeks for the cell to travel from the stratum germinativum to the stratum corneum	True ☐ False ☐
16.	Psoriasis is an inflammation of the skin with itchy, flaky skin with red patches which may blister and bleed	True ☐ False ☐
17.	Lentigo is also known as butterfly mask	True ☐ False ☐

18.	A boil is a bacterial infection	True ☐ False ☐
19.	Fibroblasts and mast cells are found in the dermis	True ☐ False ☐
20.	The dermis is made up of adipose tissue	True ☐ False ☐
21.	Sweat and sebum mix together to form a film on the surface of the skin called the acid mantle	True ☐ False ☐
22.	The UV rays in sunlight penetrate the layers of skin, converting the chemical ergosterol into Vitamin D	True ☐ False ☐
23.	Herpes zoster is a viral infection describing cold sores	True ☐ False ☐
24.	Collagen keeps the skin supple and elastic	True ☐ False ☐
25.	The stratum lucidum is known as the granular layer of the epidermis	True ☐ False ☐
26.	Folliculitis is a bacterial infection of the hair follicle and sebaceous glands	True ☐ False ☐
27.	Vasodilation occurs when the body becomes cold	True ☐ False ☐

28.	Sebum is a fatty substance produced by sebaceous glands	True ☐ False ☐
29.	The papillary layer of the dermis contains nerve endings, blood vessels and lymphatic capillaries	True ☐ False ☐
30.	The subcutaneous layer of the skin is situated below the epidermis	True ☐ False ☐
31.	People with dry skin would suffer with couperose skin	True ☐ False ☐
32.	Body odour is produced when the sweat from eccrine glands is broken down by bacteria	True ☐ False ☐
33.	Milia are produced when the sebum becomes trapped in the hair follicle with no surface opening	True ☐ False ☐
34.	Certain medications and essential oils can penetrate the layers of the skin	True ☐ False ☐
35.	Keratinisation occurs when the cells are living with a nucleus	True ☐ False ☐
36.	Mast cells secrete histamine	True ☐ False ☐
37.	Tinea corporis is another term for ringworm	True ☐ False ☐

38.	A papule is a small elevation on the skin containing pus	True ☐ False ☐
39.	A dry skin lacks oil and a dehydrated skin lacks moisture	True ☐ False ☐
40.	Sensation is a function of the skin	True ☐ False ☐
41.	Mitotic activity occurs in the matrix of the hair	True ☐ False ☐
42.	Paronychia describes the forward growth of the cuticle	True ☐ False ☐
43.	Onychorrhexis is the term given to ingrown toe nails	True ☐ False ☐
44.	Anagen is the growing stage of the hair	True ☐ False ☐
45.	The cortex is the outer layer of the hair	True ☐ False ☐
46.	Vellus hair is found all over the face and body	True ☐ False ☐
47.	The connective tissue sheath supplies the hair and follicle with blood and nerves	True ☐ False ☐

48.	The eponychium is the cuticle found under the free edge	True ☐ False ☐
49.	Koilonychia is the term used to describe spoon shaped nails	True ☐ False ☐
50.	The subcutaneous layer is located above the dermis	True ☐ False ☐

Exercise 2

Match what category of infection the following disease and disorders of the skin fall under. Please choose your answers from the box at the end of this exercise.

1.	Dermatosis Papulosa Nigra	☐ Bacterial ☐ Fungal ☐ Pigmentation	☐ Inflammatory ☐ Infestation ☐ Viral
2.	Boil	☐ Bacterial ☐ Fungal ☐ Pigmentation	☐ Inflammatory ☐ Infestation ☐ Viral
3.	Chloasma	☐ Bacterial ☐ Fungal ☐ Pigmentation	☐ Inflammatory ☐ Infestation ☐ Viral
4.	Acne Vulgaris	☐ Bacterial ☐ Fungal ☐ Pigmentation	☐ Inflammatory ☐ Infestation ☐ Viral
5.	Naevae	☐ Bacterial ☐ Fungal ☐ Pigmentation	☐ Inflammatory ☐ Infestation ☐ Viral
6.	Carbuncles	☐ Bacterial ☐ Fungal ☐ Pigmentation	☐ Inflammatory ☐ Infestation ☐ Viral
7.	Tinea Corporis	☐ Bacterial ☐ Fungal ☐ Pigmentation	☐ Inflammatory ☐ Infestation ☐ Viral
8.	Impetigo	☐ Bacterial ☐ Fungal ☐ Pigmentation	☐ Inflammatory ☐ Infestation ☐ Viral
9.	Scabies	☐ Bacterial ☐ Fungal ☐ Pigmentation	☐ Inflammatory ☐ Infestation ☐ Viral
10.	Herpes Simplex	☐ Bacterial ☐ Fungal ☐ Pigmentation	☐ Inflammatory ☐ Infestation ☐ Viral
11.	Ephelides	☐ Bacterial ☐ Fungal ☐ Pigmentation	☐ Inflammatory ☐ Infestation ☐ Viral
12.	Folliculitis	☐ Bacterial ☐ Fungal ☐ Pigmentation	☐ Inflammatory ☐ Infestation ☐ Viral

13.	Lentigo	☐ Bacterial ☐ Fungal ☐ Pigmentation	☐ Inflammatory ☐ Infestation ☐ Viral
14.	Eczema	☐ Bacterial ☐ Fungal ☐ Pigmentation	☐ Inflammatory ☐ Infestation ☐ Viral
15.	Vitiligo	☐ Bacterial ☐ Fungal ☐ Pigmentation	☐ Inflammatory ☐ Infestation ☐ Viral
16.	Tinea Pedis	☐ Bacterial ☐ Fungal ☐ Pigmentation	☐ Inflammatory ☐ Infestation ☐ Viral
17.	Herpes Zoster	☐ Bacterial ☐ Fungal ☐ Pigmentation	☐ Inflammatory ☐ Infestation ☐ Viral
18.	Dermatitis	☐ Bacterial ☐ Fungal ☐ Pigmentation	☐ Inflammatory ☐ Infestation ☐ Viral
19.	Papilloma	☐ Bacterial ☐ Fungal ☐ Pigmentation	☐ Inflammatory ☐ Infestation ☐ Viral
20.	Verruca	☐ Bacterial ☐ Fungal ☐ Pigmentation	☐ Inflammatory ☐ Infestation ☐ Viral
21.	Psoriasis	☐ Bacterial ☐ Fungal ☐ Pigmentation	☐ Inflammatory ☐ Infestation ☐ Viral
22.	Albinism	☐ Bacterial ☐ Fungal ☐ Pigmentation	☐ Inflammatory ☐ Infestation ☐ Viral
23.	Pediculosis	☐ Bacterial ☐ Fungal ☐ Pigmentation	☐ Inflammatory ☐ Infestation ☐ Viral

Exercise 3

Complete the following crosswords on The Skin, Hair & Nails by answering the clues below.

Crossword 1

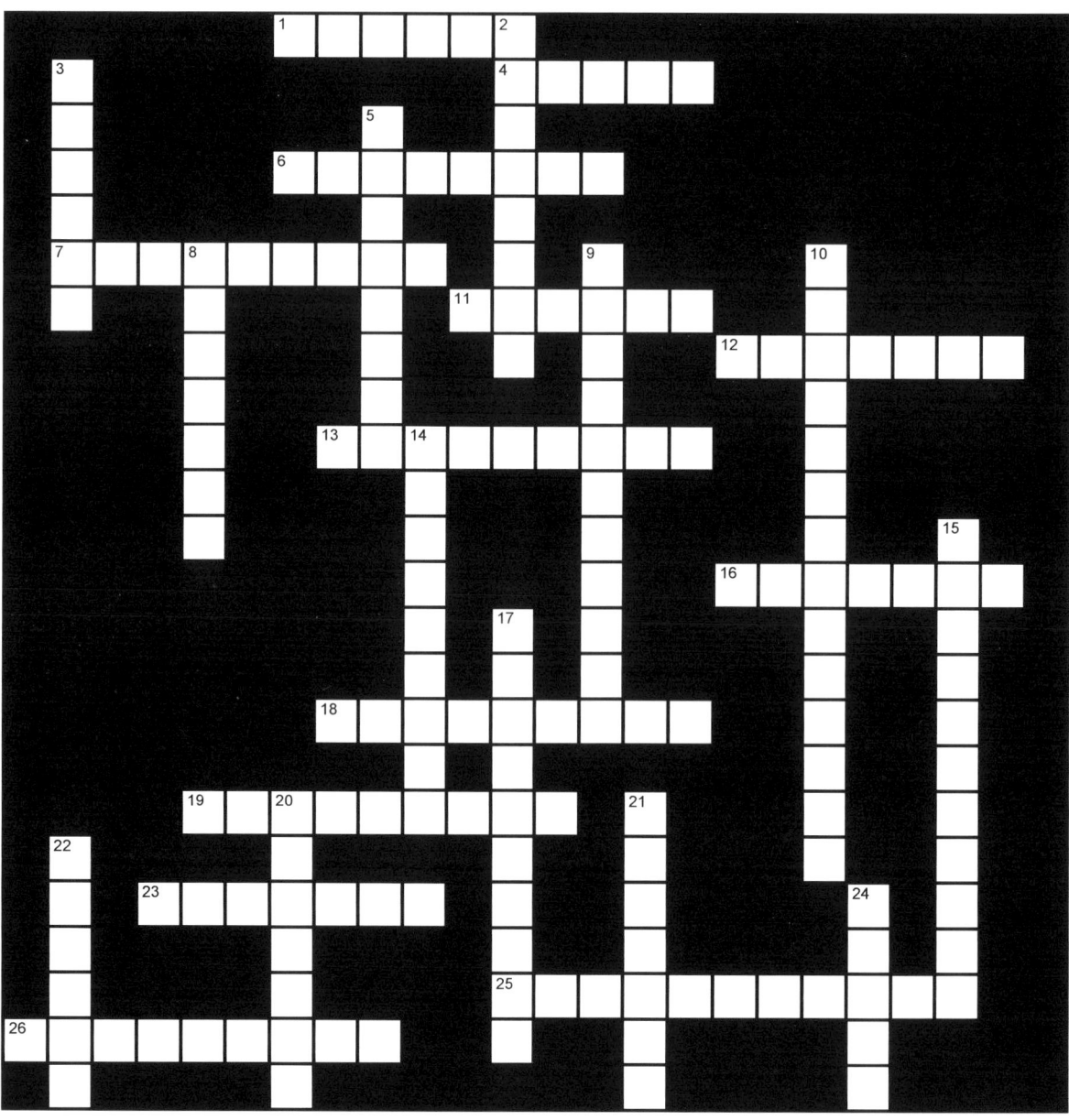

Across

1. What is the inner layer of the skin? (6)
4. What is the condition urticaria also known as? (5)
6. What type of hairs are longer and more coarse? (8)
7. Small areas of pigmented skin that appear on the skin after sun exposure (9)

11. An overgrowth of tissue of an existing healed injury (6)
12. What protein is found in the epidermis of the skin, hair and nails? (7)
13. Glands that produce an oily substance called sebum (9)
16. What substance is responsible for the colour of the skin and hair? (7)
18. What section of the hair lies above the surface of the skin? (9)
19. What layer of the skin brings vital oxygen and nutrients to the epidermis? (9)
23. What protein gives skin its elasticity? (7)
25. What term is used to describe the detachment of the nail from the nail bed? (11)
26. What layer of the skin contains mast cells and fibroblasts? (9)

Down
2. What type of viral infection affects the nerves and is highly contagious? (8)
3. During what stage of hair growth is the hair actively growing? (6)
5. The end of the nail plate, that is filed (8)
8. What type of sweat glands regulate body temperature? (7)
9. Spoon shaped nails (11)
10. What is the clear layer of the epidermis called? (14)
14. What type of infection is a carbuncle? (9)
15. What type of cells synthesize collagen fibres? (11)
17. A function of the skin (10)
20. What skin condition is commonly found on oily skin? (7)
21. What layer of the hair gives the hair its elasticity? (7)
22. The middle layer of the hair (6)
24. What layer of the epidermis separates the epidermis from the dermis? (5)

Crossword 2

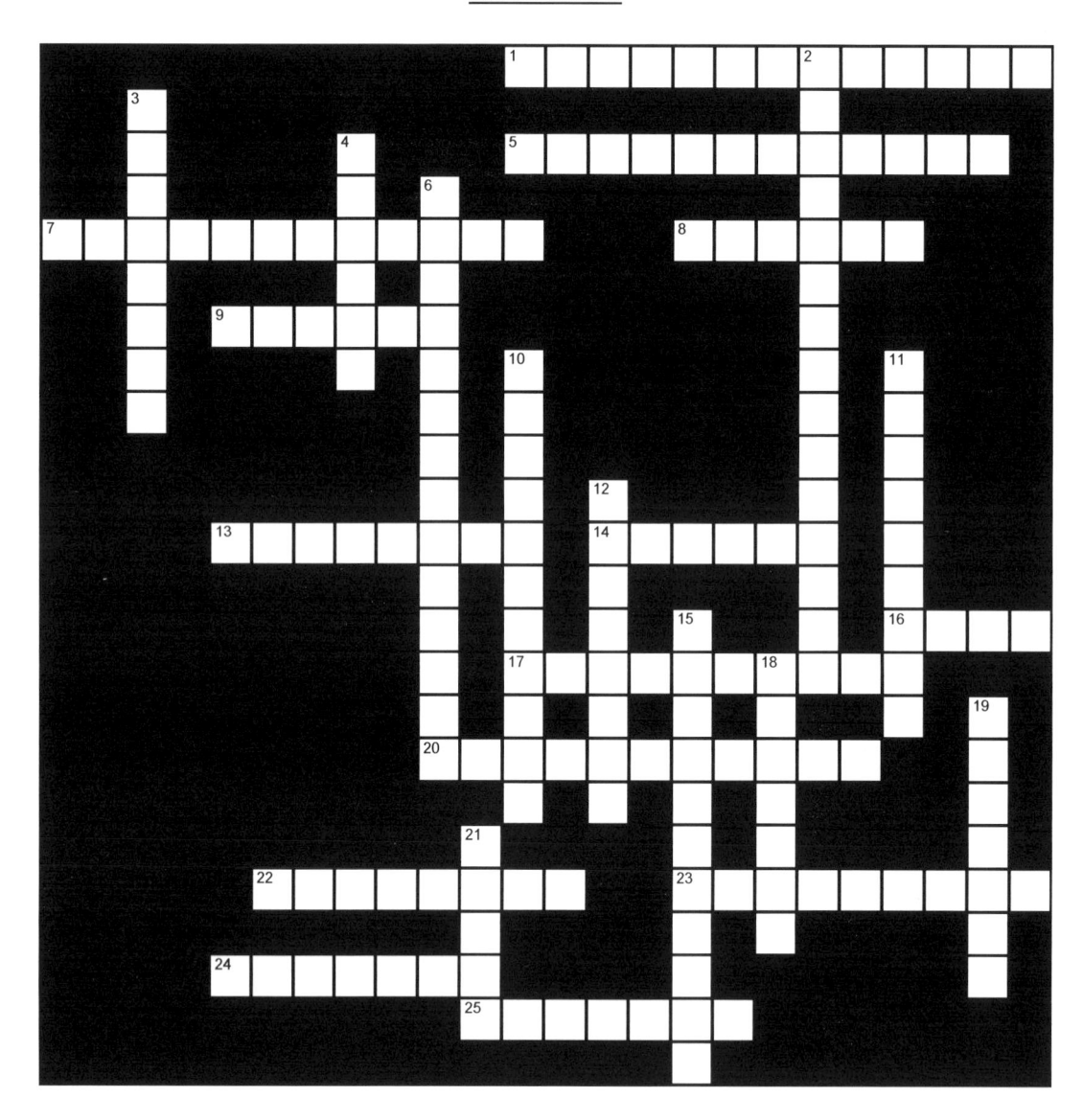

Across

1. What term is used to describe cold sores? (13)
5. What is the deepest layer of the skin and contains areolar and adipose tissue? (12)
7. A bacterial infection of the sebaceous gland and hair follicle (12)
8. What surrounds the dermal papilla? (6)
9. What is the white crescent half moon shape found at the end of the nail bed where the cuticle meets the nail? (6)
13. What part of the hair is found below the surface of the skin? (8)
14. A small, solid elevation of the skin containing no pus (6)
16. Pediculosis (4)
17. Inflammation of the skin around the nail (10)
20. What cells produce melanin? (11)

22. What condition is caused by the absence of pigmentation in the skin, hair and eyes? (8)
23. Forward growth of the cuticle on the nail bed (9)
24. What layer of the hair is responsible for the colour and sheen of hair? (7)
25. Liver spots (7)

Down
2. What do the henle's layer, huxley's layer and the cuticle form? (15)
3. What protein gives the skin its firmness and strength? (8)
4. What type of hair is soft and fine and found all over the face and body? (6)
6. What layer of the epidermis contains flat, dead, keratinised cells? (14)
10. What muscle is responsible for making the hair stand erect? (11)
11. What layer of the dermis contains collagen and elastin fibres? (9)
12. What sweat glands cause body odour? (8)
15. Nail biting (11)
18. During what stage of hair growth does the hair separate from the dermal papilla? (7)
19. A tear in the skin which often leads to cracked skin (7)
21. What type of skin infection is a verruca? (5)

Exercise 4:

In the table below, match the name of the disorder with its more commonly used name. Please choose your answers from the box at the end of this exercise.

1.	Ephelides	
2.	Erythema	
3.	Onychogryphosis	
4.	Herpes Zoster	
5.	Urticaria	
6.	Onychophagy	
7.	Pediculosis	
8.	Tinea Pedis	
9.	Pterygium	
10.	Chloasma	
11.	Milia	
12.	Leuconychia	
13	Lentigo	

Anatomy & Physiology Student Workbook

14.	Tinea Corporis	
15.	Herpes Simplex	
16.	Koilonychia	
17.	Comedones	

Please choose your answers from this grid

Freckles	Reddening of Skin	White Spots on Nails
Hives	Whiteheads	Liver Spots
Nail Biting	Blackheads	Ringworm
Shingles	Cold Sore	Overgrowth of Cuticle
Lice	Spoon Shaped Nails	Butterfly Mask
Athlete's Foot	Ingrown Nails	

Exercise 5

Please answer the questions below and find the answers in the word search puzzle.

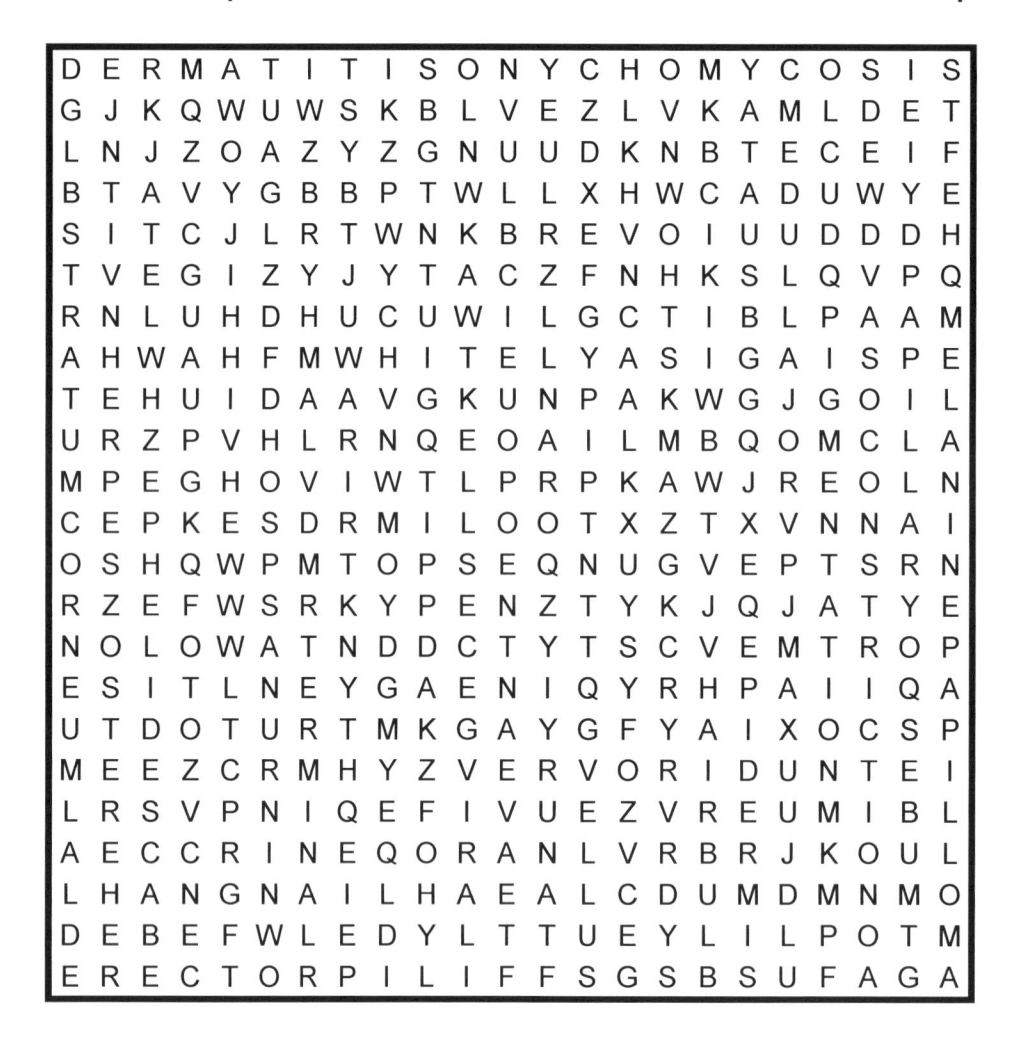

```
D E R M A T I T I S O N Y C H O M Y C O S I S
G J K Q W U W S K B L V E Z L V K A M L D E T
L N J Z O A Z Y Z G N U U D K N B T E C E I F
B T A V Y G B B P T W L L X H W C A D U W Y E
S I T C J L R T W N K B R E V O I U U D D D H
T V E G I Z Y J Y T A C Z F N H K S L Q V P Q
R N L U H D H U C U W I L G C T I B L P A A M
A H W A H F M W H I T E L Y A S I G A I S P E
T E H U I D A A V G K U N P A K W G J G O I L
U R Z P V H L R N Q E O A I L M B Q O M C L A
M P E G H O V I W T L P R P K A W J R E O L N
C E P K E S D R M I L O O T X Z T X V N N A I
O S H Q W P M T O P S E Q N U G V E P T S R N
R Z E F W S R K Y P E N Z T Y K J Q J A T Y E
N O L O W A T N D D C T Y T S C V E M T R O P
E S I T L N E Y G A E N I Q Y R H P A I I Q A
U T D O T U R T M K G A Y G F Y A I X O C S P
M E E Z C R M H Y Z V E R V O R I D U N T E I
L R S V P N I Q E F I V U E Z V R E U M I B L
A E C C R I N E Q O R A N L V R B R J K O U L
L H A N G N A I L H A E A L C D U M D M N M O
D E B E F W L E D Y L T T U E Y L I L P O T M
E R E C T O R P I L I F F S G S B S U F A G A
```

1. What is the layer of skin that we can see? (9)
2. What pigment gives skin its natural colour? (7)
3. Skin disorder characterised by red, itchy patches covered with white or silvery scales (9)
4. What is the adult form of chicken pox called? (12)
5. What is soft, fine hair found on the face and most of the body? (6)
6. What is another term used to describe a birth mark? (6)
7. What is the dead cuticle that attaches to the nail plate and grows with the nail plate as it moves upwards? (10)
8. What is another term for freckles? (9)
9. What is the term used to describe when the body heats itself up? (16)
10. What is the surface layer of the epidermis? (14)
11. What is the most abundant type of connective tissue found in the dermis? (7)
12. What is the enlarged part at the end of the hair follicle called? (8)

13. What layer of the dermis is connected to the deepest layer of the epidermis? (9)
14. What bacterial infection of the skin, commonly found on the face, causes blisters that weep and form a coloured crust? (8)
15. What are small muscles attached to each hair follicle? (11)
16. What is the inner layer of the hair? (7)
17. What is another term for liver spots? (7)
18. What protects the nail bed? (9)
19. What type of sweat glands excrete watery sweat? (7)
20. What type of infection is herpes simplex? (5)
21. A pigmentation disorder (9)
22. What is a common fungal infection of the nail? (13)
23. What fatty acid moisturises the skin? (5)
24. What type of skin disorder is albinism? (12)
25. What is the term used to describe spoon shaped nails? (11)
26. Sweat and Sebum mix together on the surface of the skin to form what? (10)
27. What describes a small split or tear of skin that hangs from the side of the nail plate? (8)
28. An inflammation of the skin caused by a chemical irritant (10)
29. What colour are the spots on the nail when you suffer from leuconychia? (5)

Exercise 6

Fill in the missing words

1. Onychorrhexis describes _____ nails (7)

2. Vitiligo is a _____ skin disorder (12)

3. _____ describes shedding of the skin (12)

4. Tinea corporis is another term used to describe _____ (8)

5. The _____ layer of the skin contains collagen and elastin fibres (9)

6. Comedones are another term used to describe _____ (10)

7. The _____ is the outer layer of the hair (7)

8. The Stratum _____ is also known as the basal layer of the epidermis (12)

9. _____ describes when a nail separates from the nail bed (11)

10. Athlete's foot is a _____ infection (6)

11. Milia are also known as _____ (10)

12. The subcutaneous layer of the skin contains fat cells that help to _____ heat loss (6)

13. Paronychia describes _____ of the skin surrounding the nail (12)

14. Collagen gives the skin its _____ (8)

15. Desquamation occurs on the stratum _____ (7)

16. The _____ is located between the cuticle and the medulla (6)

17. Vitiligo occurs when the basal layer of the skin no longer produces _____ (7)

18. The _____ is a part of the cuticle that is found under the free edge of the nail (11)

19. Folliculitis occurs when the _____ _____ and sebaceous gland are infected (4,8)

20. Herpes _____ is a term used to describe cold sores (7)

Exercise 7

Put in order, the layers that make up the skin (beginning with the deepest layer)

Subcutaneous Layer
Reticular Layer
Papillary Layer
Stratum Germinativum
Stratum Spinosum
Stratum Granulosum
Stratum Lucidum
Stratum Corneum

Please choose your answers from the box below

Stratum Lucidum	Subcutaneous Layer
Reticular Layer	Stratum Granulosum
Stratum Germinativum	Stratum Corneum
Stratum Spinosum	Papillary Layer

Exercise 8

Multiple choice questions, please choose one answer from the 4 choices provided in each box.

1. Which of the following provides a source of nourishment for the hair? a) Inner root sheath b) Connective tissue sheath c) Outer root sheath d) Erector pili muscle Answer: A	**2. What part of the hair is responsible for making the hair stand upright when we are cold?** a) Erector pili muscle b) Dermal papilla c) Apocrine gland d) Inner root sheath Answer:
3. What layer of the epidermis contains dead, flat, keratinised cells? a) Prickle cell layer b) Stratum germinativum c) Stratum corneum d) Stratum spinosum Answer:	**4. What layer of the dermis contains collagen fibres?** a) Corneum b) Granular c) Papillary d) Reticular Answer:
5. What cells found within the dermis destroy harmful wastes and bacteria? a) Mast cells b) Phagocytes c) Fibroblasts c) Histiocytes Answer:	**6. Which one of the following disorders of the skin would be aggravated by spicy food?** a) Acne rosacea b) Acne vulgaris c) Folliculitis d) Herpes simplex Answer:
7. What is the term used to describe when living cells change to dead cells? a) Ossification b) Cell regeneration c) Keratinisation d) Mitosis Answer:	**8. Which of the following is a function of keratin?** a) To provide nourishment b) To provide a blood supply c) To eliminate wastes d) To provide protection Answer:

9. What happens to the blood capillaries when the body is cold? a) They contract b) They dilate c) They become wider d) They stretch Answer:	10. During vasodilation, what helps to cool the body? a) The body hair stands on end b) Sweat evaporates on the skin's surface c) Shivering d) Blood capillaries contract Answer:
11. What helps to protect the deeper layers of the skin from UV damage? a) Keratin b) Melanin c) Sebum d) Lactic acid Answer:	12. What layer of the epidermis has fully keratinised cells? a) Stratum germinativum b) Stratum granulosum c) Stratum corneum d) Stratum spinosum Answer:
13. What type of skin disorder does dermatosis papulosa nigra fall under? a) Pigmentation b) Bacterial c) Viral d) Fungal Answer:	14. Define keloid scars; a) An overgrowth of tissue on an existing scar b) A mark remaining on the skin after an injury c) A growth on the skin which is pigmented d) A round smooth lump of tissue on the skin Answer:
15. Stretch marks are also known as; a) Cellulitis b) Striae c) Macules d) Fissure Answer:	16. An abnormal sac, found on the skin, that may contain fluid or a semi solid material; a) Papule b) Macule c) Fissure d) Cyst Answer:

17. Which one of the following is a bacterial infection? a) Carbuncle b) Herpes simplex c) Pediculosis d) Ringworm Answer:	18. Which one of the following is an infestation disorder of the skin? a) Ringworm b) Pediculosis c) Athlete's foot d) Acne rosacea Answer:
19. What is the condition called when the nail is dry, lacks moisture and splits? a) Onychogryphosis b) Onychomycosis c) Onycholysis d) Onychorrhexis Answer:	20. Which of the following is an appendage of the skin? a) Dermis b) Medulla c) Hair d) Epidermis Answer:
21. What layer of the hair determines the colour and sheen of the hair? a) Medulla b) Anagen c) Hair shaft d) Hair bulb Answer:	22. Which one of the following is not a layer of the skin? a) Dermis b) Catagen c) Epidermis d) Subcutaneous Answer:
23. The prickle cell layer is also known as; a) Stratum corneum b) Stratum lucidum c) Stratum spinosum d) Stratum germinativum Answer:	24. Which one of the following helps to warm the body when it is cold? a) Vasodilation b) Dilation of blood capillaries c) Sweating d) Shivering Answer:

25. What substance acts as the skin's natural moisturiser? a) Sebum b) Collagen c) Elastin d) Sweat Answer:	**26. Which one of the following is not a bacterial skin infection?** a) Carbuncle b) Folliculitis c) Verruca d) Impetigo Answer:
27. Which one of the following nail disorders is highly contagious? a) Onychomycosis b) Onychophagy c) Paronychia d) Onychogryphosis Answer:	**28. Which of the following is a function of the skin?** a) Heat production b) Movement c) Excretion d) Storage Answer:
29. What type of tissue is the subcutaneous layer made up of? a) Adipose and yellow elastic b) Areolar and adipose c) Areolar and lymphoid d) Adipose and fibrous Answer:	**30. What part of the nail prevents bacteria from entering the matrix?** a) Nail walls b) Nail grooves c) Lunula d) Cuticle Answer:
31. What layer of the epidermis contains melanocytes? a) Clear layer b) Prickle cell layer c) Granular layer d) Basal layer Answer:	**32. What skin disorder is caused by skin cells that reproduce very quickly?** a) Eczema b) Acne vulgaris c) Psoriasis d) Skin tags Answer:

33. Taking the contraceptive pill may cause what skin condition? a) Chloasma b) Vitiligo c) Lentigo d) Ephelides Answer:	**34. What type of hair is found under the arms?** a) Lanugo b) Vellus c) Cortex d) Terminal Answer:
35. Tinea corporis is also known as; a) Scabies b) Ringworm c) Athlete's foot d) Shingles Answer:	**36. Where on the body is the skin at its thinnest?** a) Eyelids b) Nose c) Upper lip d) Soles of the feet Answer:
37. What provides nutrients to the hair? a) Dermal papilla b) Erector pili muscle c) Medulla d) Hair bulb Answer:	**38. What pigmentation disorder causes the irises of the eyes to be pink in colour?** a) Chloasma b) Vitiligo c) Albinism d) Papilloma Answer:
39. What is the resting stage of hair growth? a) Pathogen b) Telogen c) Catagen d) Anagen Answer:	**40. What maintains the PH level of the skin?** a) Erector pili muscle b) Eccrine glands c) Sebaceous glands d) Acid mantle Answer:

The Skin, Hair & Nails

Answers

Exercise 1 (true/false):

1. True	11. True	21. True	31. False	41. True
2. False	12. False	22. True	32. False	42. False
3. True	13. False	23. False	33. True	43. False
4. True	14. True	24. False	34. True	44. True
5. False	15. False	25. False	35. False	45. False
6. False	16. False	26. True	36. True	46. True
7. True	17. False	27. False	37. True	47. True
8. False	18. True	28. True	38. False	48. False
9. True	19. True	29. True	39. True	49. True
10. True	20. False	30. False	40. True	50. False

Exercise 2 (match skin disease/disorders with the category it falls under):

1. Pigmentation
2. Bacterial
3. Pigmentation
4. Bacterial
5. Pigmentation
6. Bacterial
7. Fungal
8. Bacterial
9. Infestation
10. Viral
11. Pigmentation
12. Bacterial
13. Pigmentation
14. Inflammatory
15. Pigmentation
16. Fungal
17. Viral
18. Inflammatory
19. Pigmentation
20. Viral
21. Inflammatory
22. Pigmentation
23. Infestation

Anatomy & Physiology Student Workbook

Exercise 3 (crossword):

Crossword 1

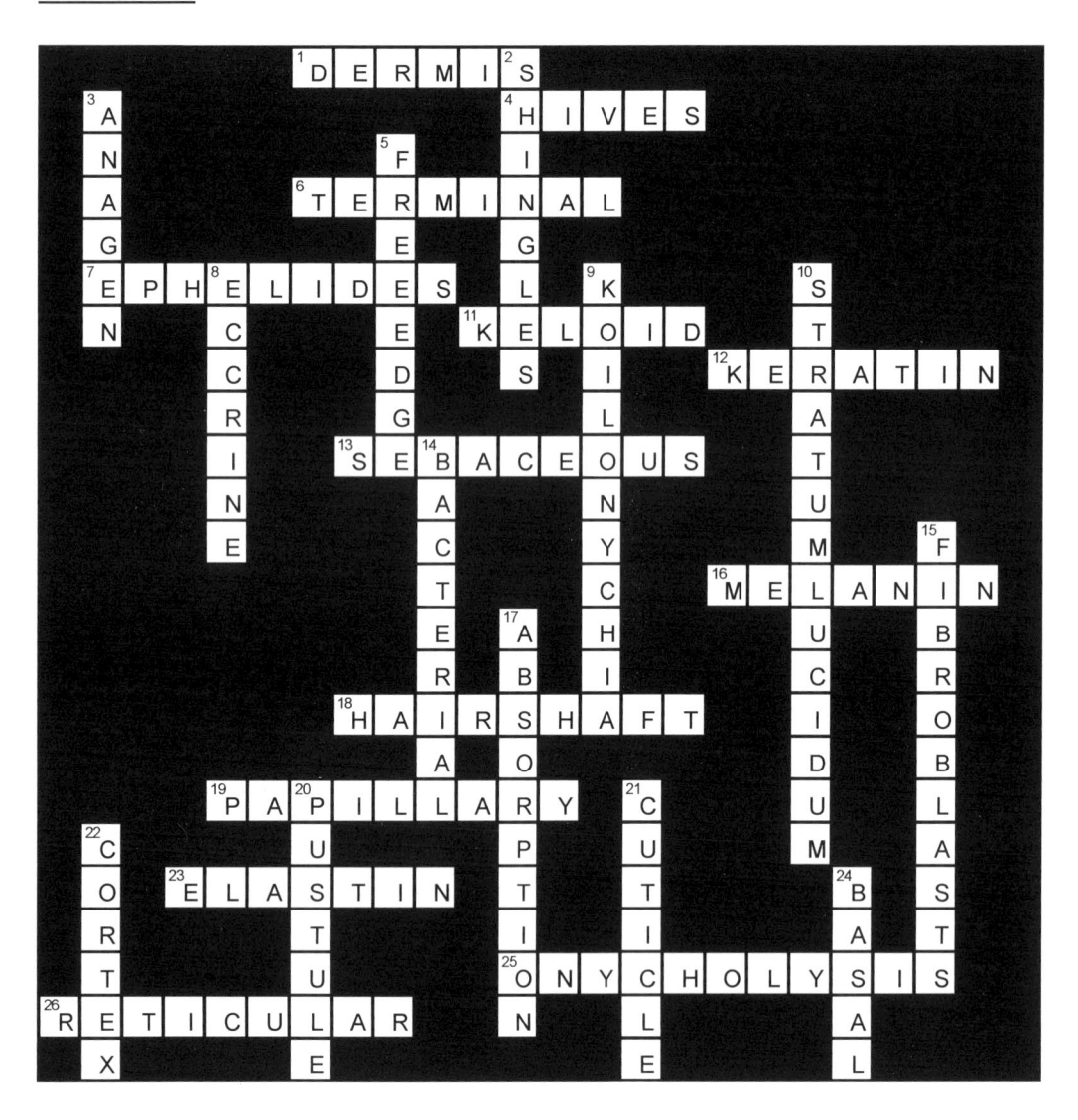

Crossword 2

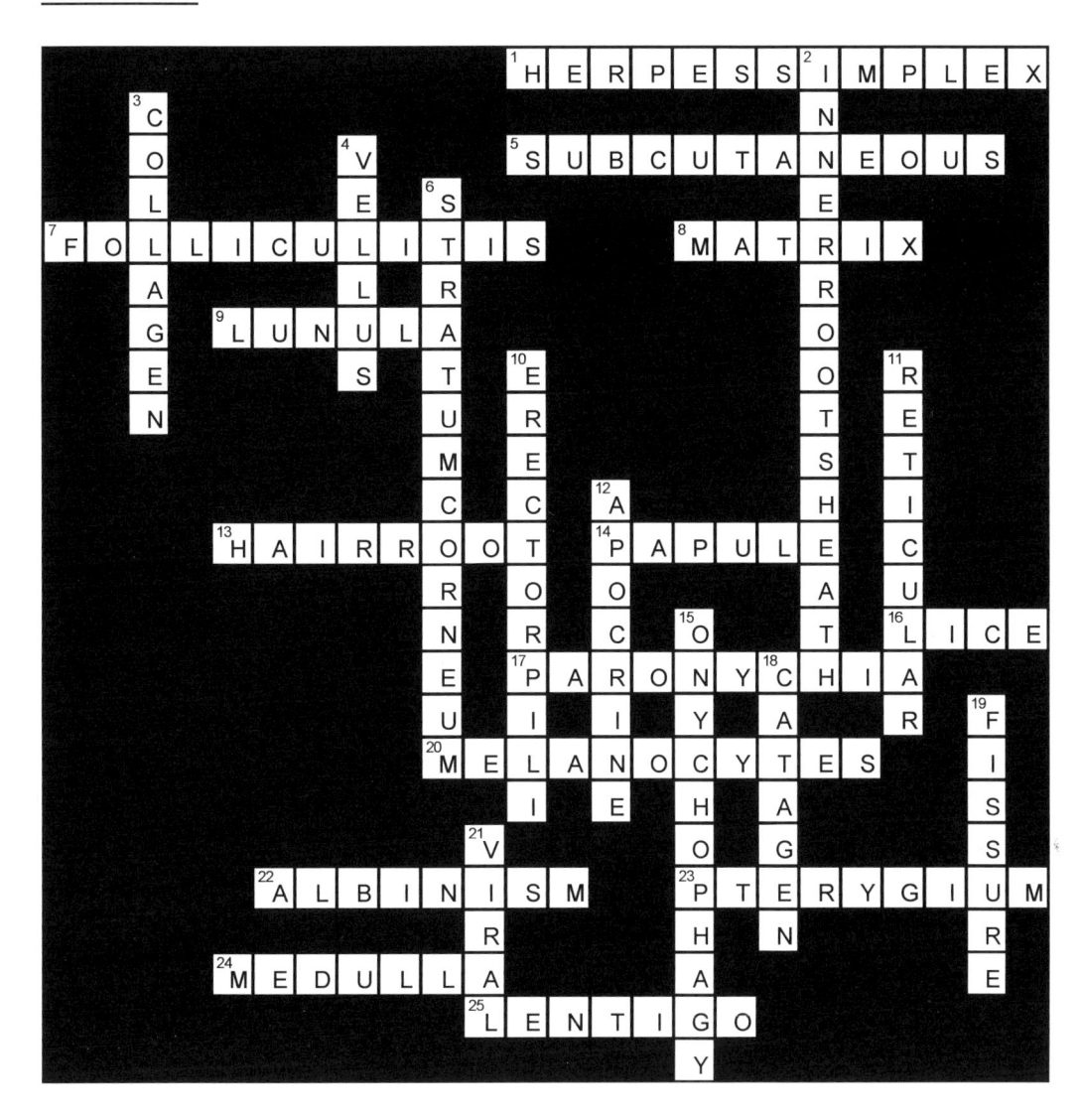

Across and down entries visible in the grid:

- 1. HERPES SIMPLEX
- 3. COLLAGEN
- 4. VELLUS
- 5. SUBCUTANEOUS
- 6. STRATUM CORNEUM
- 7. FOLLICULITIS
- 8. MATRIX
- 9. LUNULA
- 10. ERECTOR
- 11. RETICULAR
- 12. APOCRINE
- 13. HAIR ROOT
- 14. PAPULE
- 15. OCCIPITAL
- 16. LICE
- 17. PARONYCHIA
- 18. CHAR...
- 19. FISSURE
- 20. MELANOCYTES
- 21. VERRUCA
- 22. ALBINISM
- 23. PTERYGIUM
- 24. MEDULLA
- 25. LENTIGO

Exercise 4 (match the disorder with its more commonly used name):

1. Freckles
2. Reddening of Skin
3. Ingrown Nails
4. Shingles
5. Hives
6. Nail Biting
7. Lice
8. Athlete's Foot
9. Overgrowth of Cuticle
10. Butterfly Mask
11. Whiteheads
12. White Spots on Nail
13. Liver Spots
14. Ringworm
15. Cold Sore
16. Spoon Shaped Nails
17. Blackheads

Anatomy & Physiology Student Workbook

Exercise 5 (word search puzzle):

1. Epidermis
2. Melanin
3. Psoriasis
4. Herpes Zoster
5. Vellus
6. Naevae
7. Eponychium
8. Ephelides
9. Vasoconstriction
10. Stratum Corneum
11. Areolar
12. Hair Bulb
13. Papillary
14. Impetigo
15. Erector Pili
16. Medulla
17. Lentigo
18. Nail Plate
19. Eccrine
20. Viral
21. Papilloma
22. Onychomycosis
23. Sebum
24. Pigmentation
25. Koilonychia
26. Acid Mantle
27. Hang Nail
28. Dermatitis
29. White

Exercise 6 (fill in the missing words):

1. Brittle
2. Pigmentation
3. Desquamation
4. Ringworm
5. Reticular
6. Blackheads
7. Cuticle
8. Germinativum
9. Onycholysis
10. Fungal
11. Whiteheads
12. Reduce
13. Inflammation
14. Strength
15. Corneum
16. Cortex
17. Melanin
18. Hyponychia
19. Hair Follicle
20. Simplex

Exercise 7 (put the layers of the skin in order):

Subcutaneous Layer
Reticular Layer
Papillary Layer
Stratum Germinativum
Stratum Spinosum
Stratum Granulosum
Stratum Lucidum
Stratum Corneum

Exercise 8 (multiple choice questions):

1	B	9	A	17	A	25	A	33	A
2	A	10	B	18	B	26	C	34	D
3	C	11	B	19	D	27	A	35	B
4	D	12	C	20	C	28	C	36	A
5	B	13	A	21	A	29	B	37	A
6	A	14	A	22	B	30	D	38	C
7	C	15	B	23	C	31	D	39	B
8	D	16	D	24	D	32	C	40	D

Anatomy & Physiology Student Workbook

Chapter 3 | The Skeletal System

Revision Puzzles & Questions

Exercise 1

The following grid lists statements on the left that are either true or false. Please choose your answer on the right. All answers are provided at the end of the chapter.

1.	There are 206 bones in the adult body	True ☐ False ☐
2.	The scapula is an irregular bone	True ☐ False ☐
3.	Tendons attach bone to bone	True ☐ False ☐
4.	The navicular bone is a carpal	True ☐ False ☐
5.	Supination refers to turning the palm of the hand to face upwards	True ☐ False ☐
6.	Cartilaginous joints are freely moveable joints	True ☐ False ☐
7.	The mandible forms the lower jaw	True ☐ False ☐

8.	Haversian canals are found in compact bone	True ☐ False ☐
9.	The sternum is a type of sesamoid bone	True ☐ False ☐
10.	The vertebral column consists of 31 bones	True ☐ False ☐
11.	The radius is found in the upper arm	True ☐ False ☐
12.	Inversion refers to the soles of the feet facing outwards	True ☐ False ☐
13.	The ball & socket is a type of synovial joint	True ☐ False ☐
14.	Gout is a joint disorder that occurs when there is a build up of uric acid crystals around the joints	True ☐ False ☐
15.	Kyphosis is an increased inward curvature of the lumbar vertebrae	True ☐ False ☐
16.	Protection is a function of the skeleton	True ☐ False ☐
17.	The femur is known as the thigh bone	True ☐ False ☐

18.	The occipital bone forms the sides of the skull	True ☐ False ☐
19.	The patella is also known as the knee cap	True ☐ False ☐
20.	The triquetral is a tarsal	True ☐ False ☐
21.	The shoulder is a type of hinge joint	True ☐ False ☐
22.	Adduction describes moving a limb towards the midline of the body	True ☐ False ☐
23.	The cervical vertebrae are the vertebrae of the neck	True ☐ False ☐
24.	Carpals fall into the category of short bones	True ☐ False ☐
25.	The vomer forms part of the orbital cavity	True ☐ False ☐
26.	The clavicle is also known as the breast bone	True ☐ False ☐
27.	The ulna is found in the arm	True ☐ False ☐

28.	The ribs are a type of irregular bone	True ☐ False ☐
29.	The axial skeleton consists of the vertebral column	True ☐ False ☐
30.	The ilium, ischium and pubis form the pelvic girdle	True ☐ False ☐
31.	The carpals are the ankle bones	True ☐ False ☐
32.	Cancellous bone is found in the end of long bones	True ☐ False ☐
33.	The humerus is a type of flat bone	True ☐ False ☐
34.	The tibia is a type of long bone	True ☐ False ☐
35.	The maxilla holds the upper teeth	True ☐ False ☐
36.	Arthritis causes brittle bone disease	True ☐ False ☐
37.	A pivot joint allows rotation	True ☐ False ☐

38.	Extension describes straightening a body part so that the angle between the bones increases	True ☐ False ☐
39.	The calcaneus is the heel bone	True ☐ False ☐
40.	The fibula is known as the shin bone	True ☐ False ☐
41.	Osteocytes are mature bone cells	True ☐ False ☐
42.	The destruction of bone tissue is known as ossification	True ☐ False ☐
43.	Bone making cells are known as osteoclasts	True ☐ False ☐
44.	The anatomical term distal refers to being furthest away from the midline	True ☐ False ☐
45.	A condyloid joint allows movement in all directions	True ☐ False ☐

Exercise 2

Please match the category of bone with the names of the bones in the table below. Choose from:

1. Long Bone
2. Short Bone
3. Flat Bone
4. Irregular Bone
5. Sesamoid Bone

1.	Femur		16.	Mandible	
2.	Patella		17.	Talus	
3.	Maxilla		18.	Tibia	
4.	Navicular		19.	Cuboid	
5.	Humerus		20.	Palatine	
6.	Zygomatic		21	Occipital	
7.	Sacrum		22.	Phalanges	
8.	Sternum		23.	Ribs	
9.	Clavicle		24.	Vertebrae	
10.	Cuneiform		25.	Scapula	
11.	Triquetral		26.	Lunate	

Anatomy & Physiology Student Workbook

12.	Ulna		27.	Parietal	
13.	Ethmoid		28.	Metacarpals	
14.	Fibula		29.	Radius	
15.	Temporal		30.	Pisiform	

Exercise 3

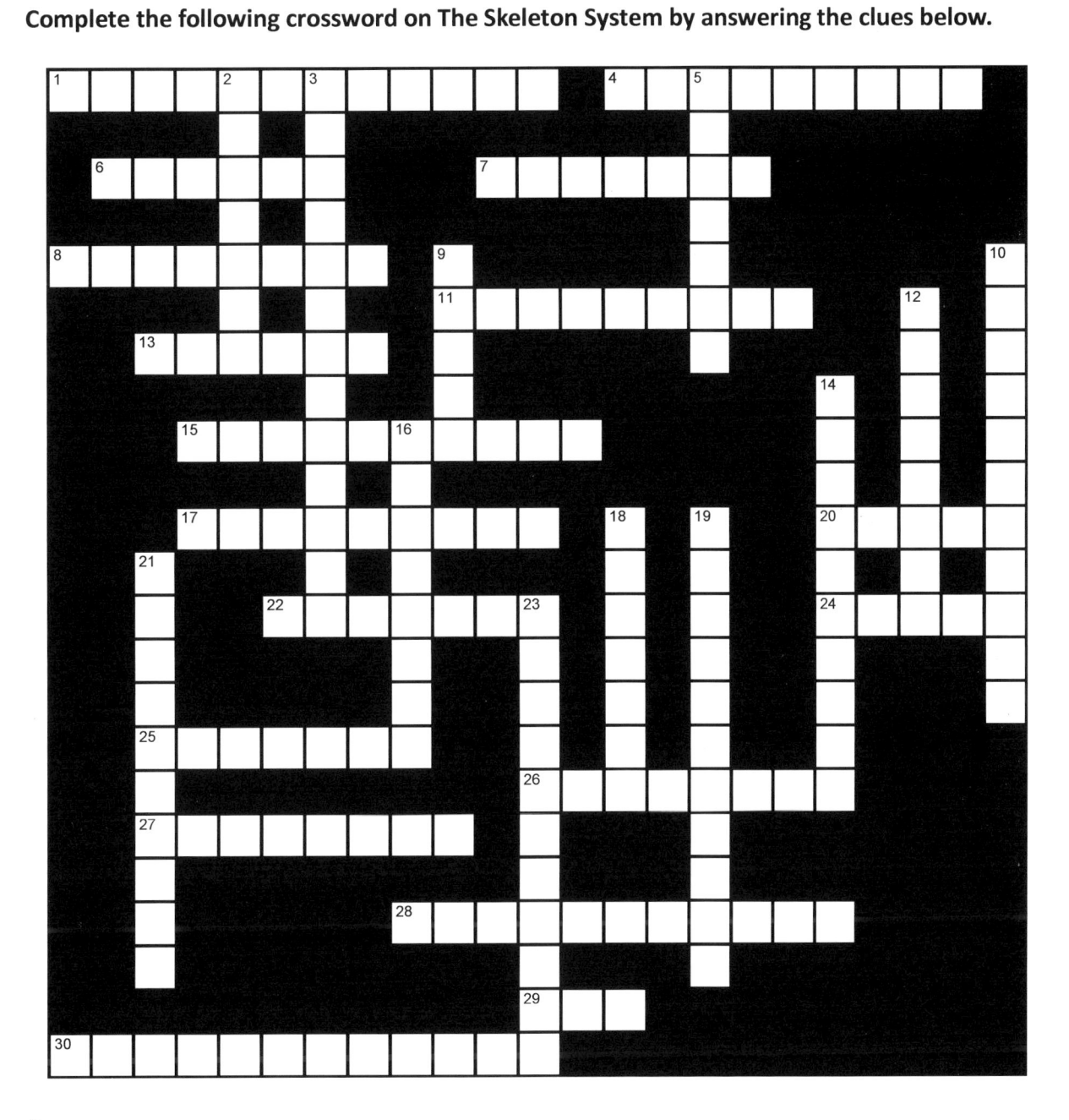

Complete the following crossword on The Skeleton System by answering the clues below.

Across
1. What is the process of bone formation called? (12)
4. What movement increases the angle between 2 bones at a joint? (9)
6. What vertebrae lie in the lower back? (6)
7. A function of the skeleton (7)
8. An increased outward curvature of the thoracic spine (8)
11. What category of bone does the maxilla fall under? (9)
13. The point furthest from the point of attachment to the body (6)

15. A membrane of connective tissue covering the surface of bones (10)
17. Cheek bone (9)
20. What part of the skeleton does the sternum belong to? (5)
22. What bone forms the lower posterior part of the pelvic girdle? (7)
24. What bone connects the leg and the foot? (5)
25. What bone forms the roof of the nasal cavity? (7)
26. Collar bone (8)
27. A tough fibrous connective tissue that connects bone to bone or bone to cartilage (8)
28. What type of fracture describes when a broken bone damages other organs or structures around it? (11)
29. What part of the body is the tibia found? (3)
30. What cells found in cartilage, help to form bone? (12)

Down
2. A fixed joint (7)
3. Slightly moveable joints (13)
5. Bones found in the ankle (7)
9. What type of joint allows rotation around an axis? (5)
10. What cells dissolve bone surfaces so that new bone can be produced? (11)
12. Freely moveable joints (8)
14. Sternum (10)
16. A carpal bone (8)
18. What type of bone falls under the category of sesamoid? (7)
19. What anatomical term describes when something is nearer to the surface? (11)
21. What type of bone tissue is light and spongy? (10)
23. Hand bones (11)

Exercise 4

In the table below, match the name of the bone with its position in the body. Please choose from the answers in the box at the end of this exercise.

1.	Cheek		14.	Thumb Side of Forearm	
2.	Thigh		15.	Side of Cranium	
3.	Fingers		16.	Lower Back	
4.	Neck		17.	Collar	
5.	Upper Arm		18.	Shoulder	
6.	Centre of Chest		19.	Medial Aspect of Lower Leg	
7.	Upper Jaw		20.	Ankle Joint	
8.	Back of Skull		21.	Little Finger Side of Forearm	
9.	Lateral Aspect of Lower Leg		22.	Roof of Mouth	
10.	Bridge of Nose		23.	Upper Sides of Cranium	
11.	Kneecap		24.	Forehead	

Anatomy & Physiology Student Workbook

12.	Pelvis			25.	Wrist Bones	
13.	Heel					

Please choose your answers from the box below

Frontal	Occipital	Humerus
Palatine	Carpals	Talus
Calcaneum	Sternum	Clavicle
Nasal	Ulna	Radius
Phalanges	Ilium	Maxilla
Femur	Cervical Vertebrae	Fibula
Zygomatic	Scapula	Lumbar Vertebrae
Tibia	Parietal	
Patella	Temporal	

Exercise 5

In the table below, please specify whether the bones are tarsals or carpals.

1.	Triquetral			8.	Navicular	
2.	Hamate			9.	Lunate	
3.	Cuneiform			10.	Pisiform	
4.	Trapezoid			11.	Scaphoid	
5.	Cuboid			12.	Calcaneus	
6.	Talus			13.	Trapezium	
7.	Capitate					

Anatomy & Physiology Student Workbook

Exercise 6

Please answer the questions below and find the answers in the word search puzzle.

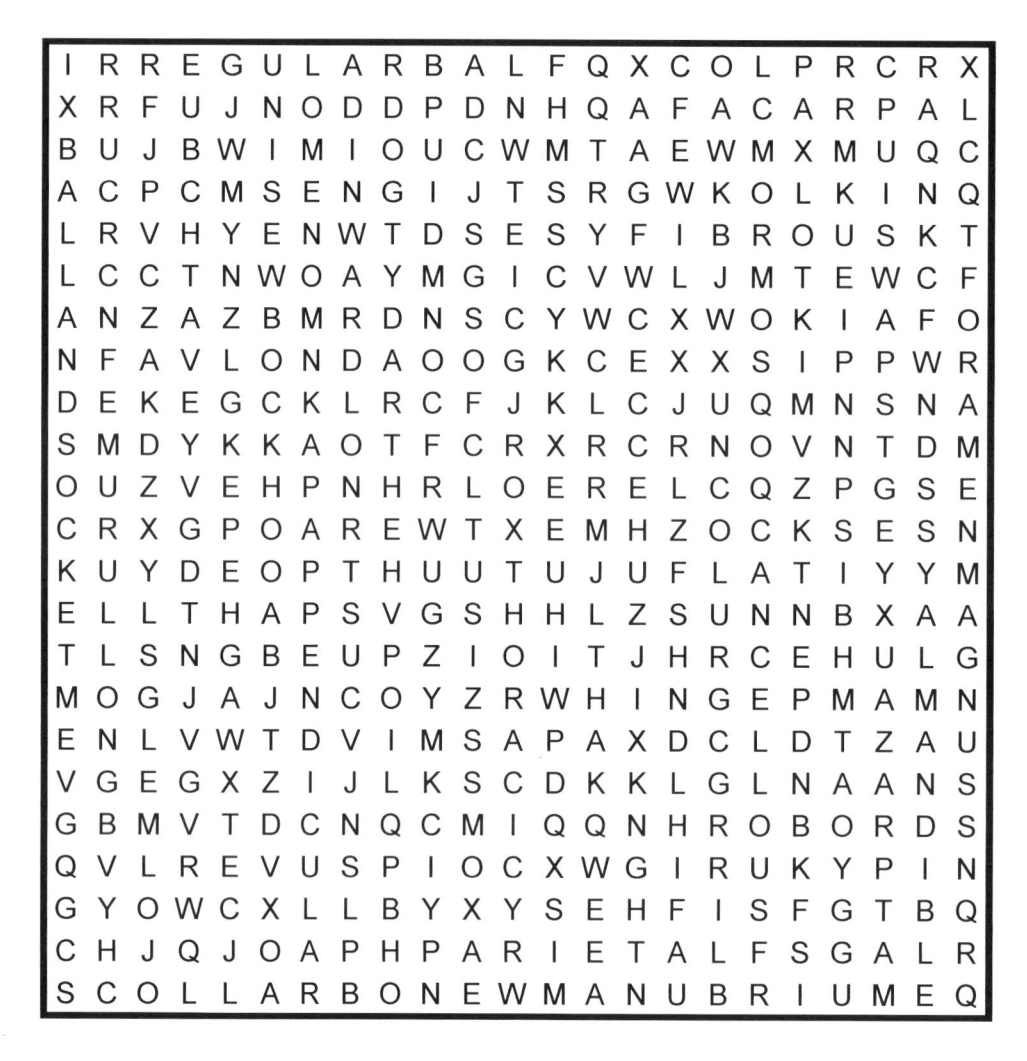

```
I R R E G U L A R B A L F Q X C O L P R C R X
X R F U J N O D D P D N H Q A F A C A R P A L
B U J B W I M I O U C W M T A E W M X M U Q C
A C P C M S E N G I J T S R G W K O L K I N Q
L R V H Y E N W T D S E S Y F I B R O U S K T
L C C T N W O A Y M G I C V W L J M T E W C F
A N Z A Z B M R D N S C Y W C X W O K I A F O
N F A V L O N D A O O G K C E X X S I P P W R
D E K E G C K L R C F J K L C J U Q M N S N A
S M D Y K K A O T F C R X R C R N O V N T D M
O U Z V E H P N H R L O E R E L C Q Z P G S E
C R X G P O A R E W T X E M H Z O C K S E S N
K U Y D E O P T H U U T J U F L A T I Y Y M
E L L T H A P S V G S H H L Z S U N N B X A A
T L S N G B E U P Z I O I T J H R C E H U L G
M O G J A J N C O Y Z R W H I N G E P M A M N
E N L V W T D V I M S A P A X D C L D T Z A U
V G E G X Z I J L K S C D K K L G L N A A N S
G B M V T D C N Q C M I Q Q N H R O B O R D S
Q V L R E V U S P I O C X W G I R U K Y P I N
G Y O W C X L L B Y X Y S E H F I S F G T B Q
C H J Q J O A P H P A R I E T A L F S G A L R
S C O L L A R B O N E W M A N U B R I U M E Q
```

1. What bone contains the lower teeth? (8)
2. What joint allows movement in one direction only? (5)
3. The ribs fall under what category of bone? (4)
4. What is the pisiform? (6)
5. What are the body's hinges? (6)
6. What part of the skeleton holds the lower limbs? (12)
7. What bone forms the top and sides of the skull? (8)
8. What is the thigh bone called? (5)
9. What type of bones are strong, cube-shaped bones that provide support and stability? (5)
10. What section of the vertebral column holds the ribs? (8)
11. What is the term used to describe brittle bone disease? (12)
12. What bone forms the forehead? (7)
13. What type of bone tissue contains bone marrow? (10)
14. What is the heel bone called? (9)

Anatomy & Physiology Student Workbook

15. What is the bone at the top of the arm called? (7)
16. What category of bone do the metacarpals fall under? (4)
17. What is the most moveable of all joints? (13)
18. What is the broad, flat upper part of the sternum called? (9)
19. A long bone of the arm (4)
20. What is another name for the clavicle? (10)
21. What part of the occipital bone does the spinal cord pass through? (13)
22. What category of bone do the vertebrae fall under? (9)
23. An irregular bone (9)
24. What is an example of a hinge joint? (5)
25. In what direction does the lower back curve when you suffer with lordosis? (6)
26. What are the finger bones called? (9)
27. What type of bone tissue contains haversian canals? (7)
28. What is an example of a sesamoid bone? (5)
29. Fixed joints (7)
30. Fused vertebrae that form the coccyx (9)

Exercise 7

In the table below, match each movement with its definition. Please choose your answers from the box at the end of this exercise.

1.	Pointing the toes down with the heel up	
2.	Turning the palm of the hand to face upwards	
3.	Moving a limb towards the midline of the body	
4.	Bending a body part to decrease the angle between the bones at a joint	
5.	Soles of the feet face outwards	
6.	Moving a limb away from the midline of the body	
7.	Turning the palm of the hand to face downwards	
8.	Soles of the feet face inwards	
9.	Bending a body part to increase the angle between the bones at a joint	
10.	Pointing the toes up and the heel down	

Please choose your answers from the box below

Plantarflexion	Inversion	Pronation
Eversion	Flexion	Dorsiflexion
Adduction	Supination	
Extension	Abduction	

Exercise 8

Fill in the missing words.

1. The maxilla is the _____ jaw bone (5)

2. Scoliosis has a _____ curvature of the spine (8)

3. The temporal bone forms the sides and _____ part of the skull (5)

4. The _____ vertebrae are located in the neck area (8)

5. _____ bones are protective with broad surfaces (4)

6. Cancellous bone is found at the ends of _____ bones (4)

7. The patella is another name for the _____ (7)

8. The shoulder blade, also called the _____ is a flat bone (7)

9. The _____ bone contains the tear ducts (8)

10. The mandible is the only _____ bone on the face (8)

11. The back of the skull is made up of the _____ bone (9)

12. _____ bones form the pelvis (10)

13. The _____ are another name for the wrist bones (7)

14. Synovial joints are _____ moveable (6)

15. Arthritis describes _____ of the joints (12)

16. The tibia is positioned on the _____ of the lower leg (6)

17. The shoulder and _____ are types of synovial joints (3)

18. There are 12 bones in the _____ vertebrae (8)

19. A _____ fracture occurs when the broken end of the bone is driven into another bone (8)

20. The humerus bone is found in the _____ arm (5)

Anatomy & Physiology Student Workbook

Exercise 9

Multiple choice questions, please choose one answer from the 4 choices provided in each box.

1. Which one of the following is not a synovial joint? a) Hinge b) Pivot c) Fibrous d) Gliding Answer	2. Ligaments attach; a) Bone to bone b) Muscle to bone c) Tendons to bone d) Fascia to muscle Answer
3. Compact bone is; a) Hard b) Soft c) Spongy d) Tissue Answer	4. Which of the following is a function of the skeleton? a) Removes carbon dioxide from the blood b) Heat production c) Helps fight infection d) Attachment for muscles Answer
5. Which bone is found in the lower leg? a) Ulna b) Femur c) Tibia d) Ilium Answer	6. The zygomatic bone is found; a) On the forehead b) On the cheek c) Lower jaw d) Behind the ear Answer
7. Which one of the following is a tarsal? a) Turbinate b) Hamate c) Capitate d) Cuboid Answer	8. What bone is positioned in the centre of the chest? a) Sternum b) Scapula c) Clavicle d) Radius Answer

9. An increased inward curvature of the lumbar spine; a) Scoliosis b) Lordosis c) Kyphosis d) Arthritis Answer	10. Which one of the following is not a type of bone? a) Irregular b) Flat c) Cartilaginous d) Long Answer
11. How many thoracic vertebrae are there? a) 5 b) 12 c) 10 d) 14 Answer	12. Which of the following is the shinbone? a) Fibula b) Femur c) Patella d) Tibia Answer
13. What is found in cancellous bone? a) Red bone marrow b) Haversian canals c) Lymphatic vessels d) Phagocytes Answer	14. Which one of the following is not a long bone? a) Metacarpals b) Carpals c) Ulna d) Femur Answer
15. Which bone forms the forehead? a) Temporal b) Parietal c) Frontal d) Occipital Answer	16. The appendicular skeleton supports; a) Skull b) Ribs c) Upper limbs d) Sternum Answer
17. Phalanges are; a) Ribs b) Ankle bones c) Wrist bones d) Finger bones Answer	18. Fibrous joints are; a) Immoveable b) Slightly moveable c) Freely moveable d) Gliding Answer

19. The vertebrae of the lower back are called;
a) Coccygeal
b) Cervical
c) Sacral
d) Lumbar

Answer _____

20. What is the function of intervertebral discs?
a) To provide nutrients
b) To absorb shock
c) To produce heat
d) To provide leverage when walking

Answer _____

21. The ribs are classified as;
a) Flat bones
b) Long bones
c) Sesamoid bones
d) Irregular bones

Answer _____

22. The pubic bones form the;
a) Ischium
b) Innominate bones
c) Ilium
d) Pubis

Answer _____

23. What joint allows movement in one direction?
a) Gliding
b) Hinge
c) Pivot
d) Saddle

Answer _____

24. What are the foot bones?
a) Metatarsals
b) Carpals
c) Tarsals
d) Metacarpals

Answer _____

25. Which of the following parts of the body are not part of the axial skeleton?
a) Vertebral column
b) Ribs
c) Shoulder girdle
d) Sternum

Answer _____

26. Which bone forms part of the nasal cavities?
a) Lacrimal
b) Ethmoid
c) Occipital
d) Sphenoid

Answer _____

27. What category of bones are developed within tendons? a) Flat b) Short c) Long d) Sesamoid Answer _____	**28. What is the largest bone in the foot?** a) Cuboid b) Talus c) Calcaneus d) Cuneiform Answer _____
29. How many cervical vertebrae are there? a) 5 b) 12 c) 7 d) 4 Answer _____	**30. What do the last 4 vertebrae form?** a) Sacrum b) Coccyx c) Pubis d) Pelvic girdle Answer _____
31. The collar bone is called the; a) Clavicle b) Manubrium c) Sternum d) Scapula Answer _____	**32. Which of the following is an irregular bone?** a) Occipital b) Humerus c) Patella d) Maxilla Answer _____
33. Which one of the following is not a carpal? a) Lunate b) Scaphoid c) Capitate d) Navicular Answer _____	**34. What type of joint is the shoulder?** a) Cartilaginous b) Ball and Socket c) Hinge d) Saddle Answer _____
35. What bone is positioned on the lateral lower leg? a) Fibula b) Tibia c) Femur d) Patella Answer _____	**36. How many vertebrae are there?** a) 33 b) 31 c) 17 d) 32 Answer _____

37. What bone is situated on the little finger side of the forearm? a) Radius b) Ulna c) Phalanges d) Humerus Answer	38. Freely moveable joints are known as; a) Fibrous b) Synovial c) Fixed d) Cartilaginous Answer
39. What is caused when a ligament is overstretched? a) Cramp b) Strain c) Gout d) Sprain Answer	40. What is the membrane called that covers bone? a) Osteoblasts b) Bone marrow c) Periosteum d) Haversian canals Answer

The Skeletal System
Answers

Exercise 1 (true/false):

1. True	11. False	21. False	31. False	41. True
2. False	12. False	22. True	32. True	42. False
3. False	13. True	23. True	33. False	43. False
4. False	14. True	24. True	34. True	44. True
5. True	15. False	25. False	35. True	45. False
6. False	16. True	26. False	36. False	
7. True	17. True	27. True	37. True	
8. True	18. False	28. False	38. True	
9. False	19. True	29. True	39. True	
10. False	20. False	30. True	40. False	

Exercise 2 (match the names of bone with their category):

1. Long	11. Short	21. Flat
2. Sesamoid	12. Long	22. Long
3. Irregular	13. Irregular	23. Flat
4. Short	14. Long	24. Irregular
5. Long	15. Flat	25. Flat
6. Irregular	16. Irregular	26. Short
7. Irregular	17. Short	27. Flat
8. Flat	18. Long	28. Long
9. Long	19. Short	29. Long
10. Short	20. Irregular	30. Short

Exercise 3 (crossword):

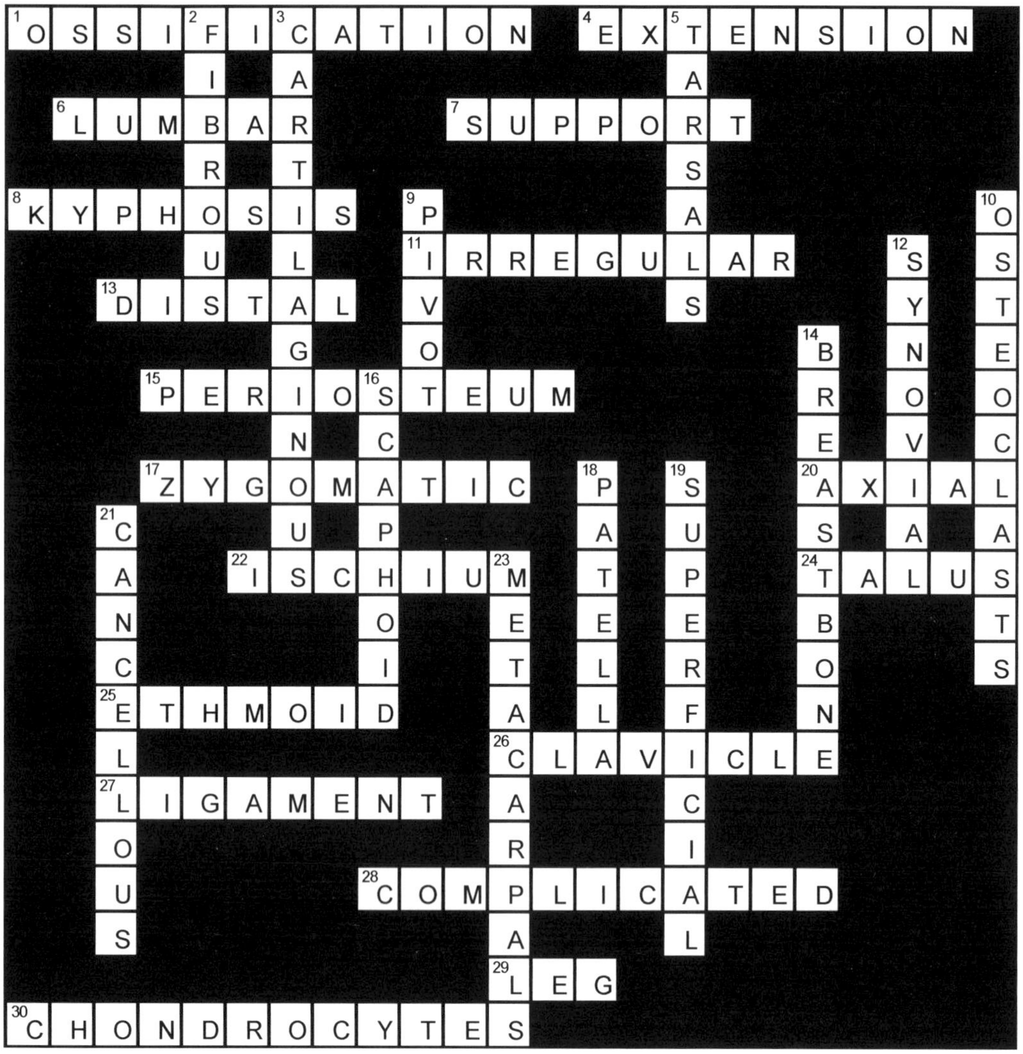

1 OSSIFICATION
4 EXTENSION
6 LUMBAR
7 SUPPORT
8 KYPHOSIS
11 IRREGULAR
13 DISTAL
15 PERIOSTEUM
17 ZYGOMATIC
20 AXIAL
22 ISCHIUM
24 TALUS
25 ETHMOID
26 CLAVICLE
27 LIGAMENT
28 COMPLICATED
29 LEG
30 CHONDROCYTES
2 FIBROUS
3 CARTILAGINOUS
5 TARSALS
9 PIVOT
10 OSTEOCLASTS
12 SYNOVIAL
14 BREASTBONE
16 SCAPHOID
18 PATELLA
19 SUPERFICIAL
21 CANCELLOUS
23 METATARSALS

Exercise 4 (match name of the bone with the position in the body):

1. Zygomatic
2. Femur
3. Phalanges
4. Cervical Vertebrae
5. Humerus
6. Sternum
7. Maxilla
8. Occipital
9. Fibula
10. Nasal
11. Patella
12. Ilium
13. Calcaneus
14. Radius
15. Temporal
16. Lumbar Vertebrae
17. Clavicle
18. Scapula
19. Tibia
20. Talus
21. Ulna
22. Palatine
23. Parietal
24. Frontal
25. Carpals

Exercise 5 (specify whether the stated bones are carpals or tarsals):

1. Carpal
2. Carpal
3. Tarsal
4. Carpal
5. Tarsal
6. Tarsal
7. Carpal
8. Tarsal
9. Carpal
10. Carpal
11. Carpal
12. Tarsal
13. Carpal

Exercise 6 (word search):

1. Mandible
2. Hinge
3. Flat
4. Carpal
5. Joints
6. Appendicular
7. Parietal
8. Femur
9. Short
10. Thoracic
11. Osteoporosis
12. Frontal
13. Cancellous
14. Calcaneus
15. Humerus
16. Long
17. Ball and Socket
18. Manubrium
19. Ulna
20. Collar Bone
21. Foramen Magnus
22. Irregular
23. Zygomatic
24. Elbow
25. Inward
26. Phalanges
27. Compact
28. Hyoid
29. Fibrous
30. Coccygeal

Anatomy & Physiology Student Workbook

Exercise 7 (match the movements with their definitions):

1. Plantarflexion
2. Supination
3. Adduction
4. Flexion
5. Eversion
6. Abduction
7. Pronation
8. Inversion
9. Extension
10. Dorsiflexion

Exercise 8 (fill in the missing words):

1. Upper
2. Sideways
3. Lower
4. Cervical
5. Flat
6. Long
7. Kneecap
8. Scapula
9. Lacrimal
10. Moveable
11. Occipital
12. Innominate
13. Carpals
14. Freely
15. Inflammation
16. Inside
17. Hip
18. Thoracic
19. Impacted
20. Upper

Exercise 9 (multiple choice questions):

1	C	9	B	17	D	25	C	33	D
2	A	10	C	18	A	26	B	34	B
3	A	11	B	19	D	27	D	35	A
4	D	12	D	20	B	28	C	36	A
5	C	13	A	21	A	29	C	37	B
6	B	14	B	22	D	30	B	38	B
7	D	15	C	23	B	31	A	39	D
8	A	16	C	24	A	32	D	40	C

Anatomy & Physiology Student Workbook

Chapter 4 | The Muscular System

Revision Puzzles & Questions

Exercise 1

The following grid lists statements on the left that are either true or false. Please choose your answer on the right. All answers are provided at the end of the chapter.

1.	The brachialis extends the forearm	True ☐ False ☐
2.	The peroneus longus plantarflexes and everts the foot	True ☐ False ☐
3.	The Sartorius flexes the knee	True ☐ False ☐
4.	The biceps femoris is part of the quadriceps group	True ☐ False ☐
5.	The masseter is the main muscle of mastication	True ☐ False ☐
6.	The latissimus dorsi laterally rotates the humerus	True ☐ False ☐
7.	The gracilis extends the knee	True ☐ False ☐

8.	The psoas muscle flexes the knee	True ☐ False ☐
9.	The subscapularis medially rotates the humerus	True ☐ False ☐
10.	The occipitalis draws the scalp forwards	True ☐ False ☐
11.	The orbicularis oculi closes the eye	True ☐ False ☐
12.	The extensor hallucis longus extends the big toe	True ☐ False ☐
13.	The pronator teres pronates the forearm	True ☐ False ☐
14.	The rhomboids adduct the scapula	True ☐ False ☐
15.	The sternocleidomastoid extends the neck	True ☐ False ☐
16.	The gracilis abducts the thigh	True ☐ False ☐
17.	The tibialis anterior dorsiflexes and inverts the foot	True ☐ False ☐

18.	The orbicularis oris opens the mouth	True ☐ False ☐
19.	The levator scapula elevates the scapula	True ☐ False ☐
20.	The coracobrachialis adducts and flexes the humerus	True ☐ False ☐
21.	The opponens digiti minimi abducts the thumb	True ☐ False ☐
22.	The soleus dorsiflexes the foot	True ☐ False ☐
23.	The erector spinae medially flexes the vertebral column	True ☐ False ☐
25.	The adductor magnus extends the hip	True ☐ False ☐
26.	The flexor carpi ulnaris flexes the wrist	True ☐ False ☐
27.	The external intercostals lift the ribcage during inhalation	True ☐ False ☐
28.	The levator labii superioris lifts the upper lip	True ☐ False ☐

29.	The flexor digiti minimi is part of the hypothenar eminence	True ☐ False ☐
30.	The flexor pollicis brevis is part of the hypothenar eminence	True ☐ False ☐
31.	Skeletal muscle is also known as voluntary muscle	True ☐ False ☐
32.	The muscles help to maintain the posture of the body	True ☐ False ☐
33.	Involuntary muscle is attached to bone	True ☐ False ☐
34.	Ligaments attach muscle to bone	True ☐ False ☐
35.	An agonist is the main muscle that is contracting	True ☐ False ☐
36.	Isotonic contraction occurs when the muscle works but does not actually move	True ☐ False ☐
37.	Eversion refers to turning the foot away from the centre	True ☐ False ☐
38.	Pronation involves turning the palm of the hand to face downwards	True ☐ False ☐

39.	Plantarflexion involves pressing the heel down and the toe up	True ☐ False ☐
39.	Plantarflexion involves pressing the heel down and the toe up	True ☐ False ☐
40.	The gastrocnemius is positioned at the side of the lower leg	True ☐ False ☐
41.	The orbicularis oculi is positioned around the mouth	True ☐ False ☐
42.	The origin of a muscle is the part that does not move	True ☐ False ☐
43.	Spasticity refers to inflammation of the muscle	True ☐ False ☐
44.	Adduction involves moving a body part towards the midline of the body	True ☐ False ☐
45.	Non striated muscle is found in the walls of the blood vessels	True ☐ False ☐
46.	The platysma is positioned at the back of the neck	True ☐ False ☐
47.	The waste product, lactic acid, is produced by the muscles after excessive exercise	True ☐ False ☐

48.	Actin and myosin are proteins found in smooth muscle	True ☐ False ☐
49.	Atrophy refers to the wasting away of the muscle	True ☐ False ☐
50.	The storage of oxygen in the muscle is a function of the muscular system	True ☐ False ☐

Exercise 2

In the table below, match the muscles of the head and neck with their corresponding actions. Please choose from the answers in the box at the end of this exercise.

1.	Draw scalp forward		11.	Raise the corners of the mouth	
2.	Closes the eye		12.	Raise lower jaw	
3.	Lower the bottom lip		13.	Lift angle of mouth up and out	
4.	Extends the head and neck		14.	Moves the mandible out	
5.	Opens and compresses nostrils		15.	Lower the corners of the mouth	
6.	Purses lips		16.	Draws scalp backwards	
7.	Lifts the mandible		17.	Compresses cheek	
8.	Raises upper lip		18.	Depresses lower jaw and lower lip	
9.	Draw the eyebrows inwards		19.	Raise and turn lower lip out	

Anatomy & Physiology Student Workbook

| 10. | Flex head and rotate head to opposite side | | | 20. | Raise lower jaw and clench teeth | |

Please choose your answers from the box below

Nasalis	Buccinator	Orbicularis Oculi
Medial Pterygoid	Temporalis	Depressor Labii Inferioris
Frontalis	Occipitalis	Sternocleidomastoid
Procerus	Platysma	Zygomaticus
Depressor Anguli Oris	Levator Labii Superioris	Orbicularis Oris
Mentalis	Lateral Pterygoid	Levator Anguli Oris
Splenius Capitis	Masseter	

Exercise 3

Complete the following crossword on The Muscular System by answering the clues below.

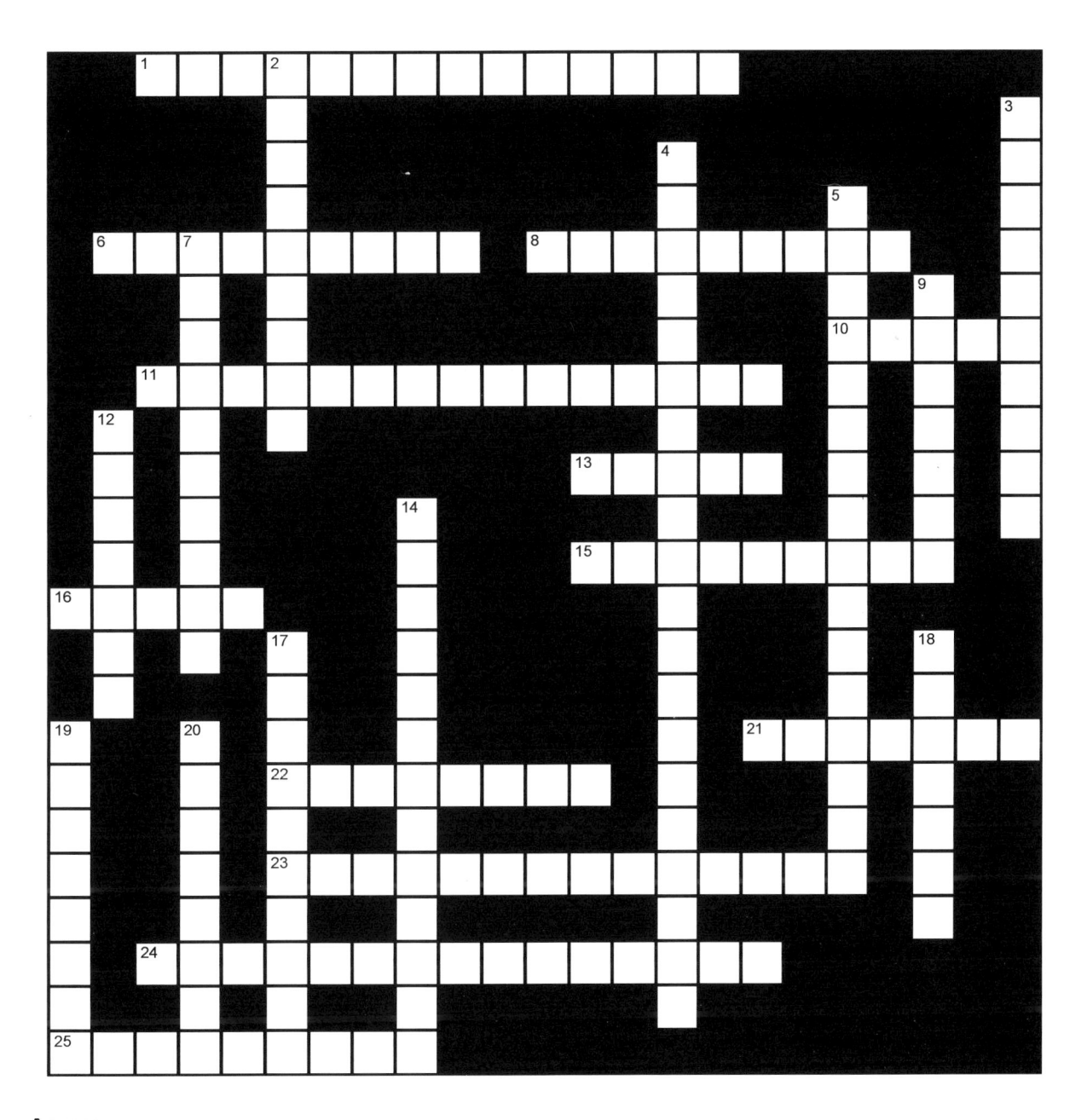

Across
1. A hamstring muscle found on top of the semimembranosus (14)
6. A triangular shaped muscle found in the upper back (9)
8. What is the most moveable point of a muscle called? (9)
10. What protein affects muscle contraction? (5)
11. What muscle extends, adducts and medially rotates the arm? (15)
13. What part of the body does the occipitalis move? (5)

Anatomy & Physiology Student Workbook — Page 93

15. What type of muscle tissue is mostly attached to bone? (9)
16. What part of the body does the flexor carpi ulnaris flex? (5)
21. What part of the body do the rhomboids adduct? (7)
22. What muscle pulls back the angle of the mouth? (8)
23. What muscle abducts and medially rotates the femur? (14)
24. What part of the body does the rectus abdominis flex? (15)
25. What muscle flexes the hip and knee? (9)

Down
2. What type of muscle contraction occurs when the muscle works by increasing tension without creating movement? (9)
3. What type of isotonic contraction occurs when the muscle shortens as it contracts? (10)
4. What muscle flexes the big toe? (20)
5. What muscle flexes and adducts the humerus? (16)
7. What is the term used to describe when 2 muscles work together by pulling in opposite directions to each other? (10)
9. What describes the wasting away of muscle tissue? (7)
12. What part of the body does the infraspinatus laterally rotate? (7)
14. What muscle crosses the front of the elbow? (13)
17. What muscle is used when frowning? (10)
18. What is required by the muscle in order to produce energy? (7)
19. Inflammation of skeletal muscle (8)
20. A function of the muscular system (8)

Exercise 4

In the table below, match the muscles of the lower limbs with their positions on the body. Please choose from the answers in the box at the end of this exercise.

1.	Medial side of thigh		11.	Front of lower leg	
2.	Inside upper thigh		12.	Front of thigh	
3.	From front of fibula to big toe		13.	From back of fibula to big toe	
4.	Back of lower leg, beneath gastrocnemius		14.	Crosses front of thigh from ilium to medial side of tibia	
5.	Outside back of thigh		15.	Front of lower leg to the toes	
6.	Outside front of thigh		16.	Medial side of the back of thigh	
7.	From back of tibia to toes		17.	Back of lower leg	
8.	Medial side of thigh underneath semitendinosus		18.	On inside of the foot	
9.	Front of thigh under rectus femoris		19.	From anterior surface of fibula to 5th metatarsal	

Anatomy & Physiology Student Workbook

| 10. | Lateral aspect of lower leg | | 20. | Back of lower leg | |

Please choose your answers from the box below

Vastus Lateralis	Extensor Hallucis Longus	Gastrocnemius
Rectus Femoris	Tibialis Anterior	Peroneus Tertius
Sartorius	Gracilis	Flexor Hallucis Longus
Adductor Brevis	Soleus	Tibialis Posterior
Vastus Intermedius	Abductor Hallucis	Extensor Digitorum Longus
Biceps Femoris	Peroneus Longus	Flexor Digitorum Longus
Semitendinosus	Semimembranosus	

Exercise 5

In the table below, match the muscles of the arms and hands with their positions in the body. Please choose from the answers in the box below.

1.	From scapula to humerus		7.	Front of upper arm	
2.	Back of forearm on ulna side		8.	Posterior forearm on radial side	
3.	Front of forearm across elbow joint		9.	Front of forearm of ulna side	
4.	Palm of hand on radial side		10.	Outside Posterior forearm	
5.	Back of upper arm		11.	Elbow	
6.	Anterior forearm on radial side		12.	Front of forearm	

Please choose your answers from the box below

Biceps	Flexor Carpi Ulnaris
Pronator Teres	Flexor Carpi Superficialis
Anconeus	Triceps
Extensor Carpi Ulnaris	Extensor Carpi Digitorum
Thenar Eminence	Flexor Carpi Radialis
Coracobrachialis	Extensor Carpi Radialis

Exercise 6

Please answer the questions below and find the answers in the word search puzzle.

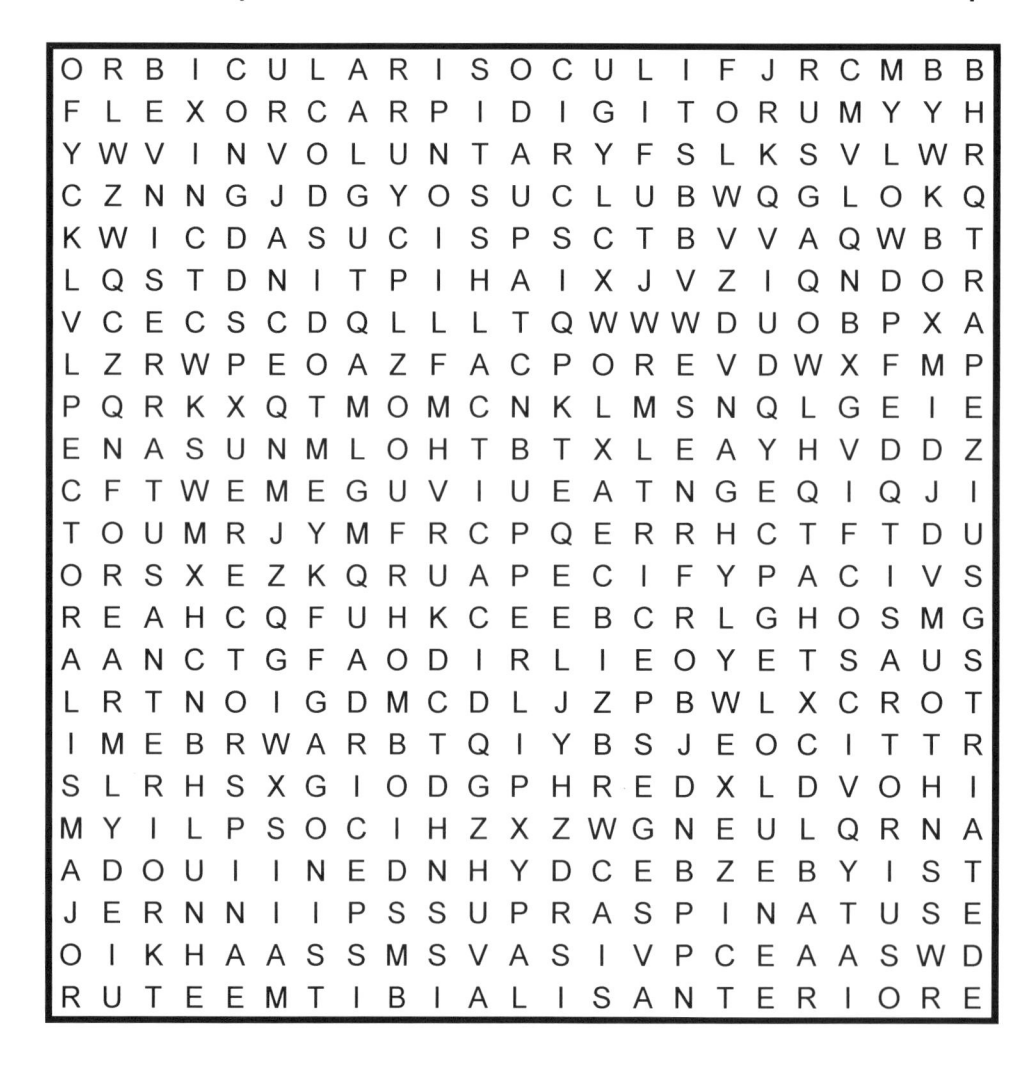

```
O R B I C U L A R I S O C U L I F J R C M B B
F L E X O R C A R P I D I G I T O R U M Y Y H
Y W V I N V O L U N T A R Y F S L K S V L W R
C Z N N G J D G Y O S U C L U B W Q G L O K Q
K W I C D A S U C I S P S C T B V V A Q W B T
L Q S T D N I T P I H A I X J V Z I Q N D O R
V C E C S C D Q L L L T Q W W W D U O B P X A
L Z R W P E O A Z F A C P O R E V D W X F M P
P Q R K X Q T M O M C N K L M S N Q L G E I E
E N A S U N M L O H T B T X L E A Y H V D D Z
C F T W E M E G U V I U E A T N G E Q I Q J I
T O U M R J Y M F R C P Q E R R H C T F T D U
O R S X E Z K Q R U A P E C I F Y P A C I V S
R E A H C Q F U H K C E E B C R L G H O S M G
A A N C T G F A O D I R L I E O Y E T S A U S
L R T N O I G D M C D L J Z P B W L X C R O T
I M E B R W A R B T Q I Y B S J E O C I T T R
S L R H S X G I O D G P H R E D X L D V O H I
M Y I L P S O C I H Z X Z W G N E U L Q R N A
A D O U I I N E D N H Y D C E B Z E B Y I S T
J E R N N I I P S S U P R A S P I N A T U S E
O I K H A A S S M S V A S I V P C E A A S W D
R U T E E M T I B I A L I S A N T E R I O R E
```

1. In what direction does the pectoralis major rotate the arm? (8)
2. What muscle flexes the fingers? (20)
3. What movement of the foot is caused by the tendon of achilles? (14)
4. What muscle commonly holds the most upper body tension? (9)
5. What muscle pulls the scapula forwards? (16)
6. What muscle turns the lower lip outwards? (8)
7. What muscle is positioned on the scapula above the spine? (13)
8. What is the main part of a muscle called? (5)
9. What muscle produces a smiling expression? (11)
10. What is another name for skeletal muscle? (8)
11. What muscle extends the elbow? (7)
12. What muscle inverts and dorsiflexes the foot? (16)
13. What part of the body is lifted by the risorius? (8)
14. What is the chest muscle called? (15)

Anatomy & Physiology Student Workbook

15. What muscle is positioned between the scapula and the spine? (9)
16. What muscle group includes the vastus lateralis? (10)
17. What muscle closes the eyelid? (16)
18. What is the shoulder muscle called? (7)
19. What waste product causes the muscles to ache? (10)
20. What is another term to describe smooth muscle? (11)
21. What body part does the supinator radii brevi turn to face upwards? (7)
22. What muscle flexes the hip and knee and laterally rotates the thigh? (9)
23. What is the main contracting muscle called? (7)
24. What connects a muscle to bone? (6)
25. What muscle is positioned either side of the spine? (13)

Exercise 7

In the table below, match the muscles of the torso with their positions on the body. Choose from the answers in the box below. Please note, some positions may be repeated.

1.	Erector Spinae		11.	Internal obliques	
2.	Pectoralis Major		12.	Infraspinatus	
3.	Latissimus Dorsi		13.	Trapezius	
4.	Rectus Abdominis		14.	Teres Major	
5.	Psoas		15.	Deltoid	
6.	Gluteus Maximus		16.	External Obliques	
7.	Supraspinatus		17.	Iliacus	
8.	Serratus Anterior		18.	Gluteus Medius	
9.	Rhomboids		19.	Transverse Abdominus	
10.	Teres Minor		20.	Supraspinatus	

Anatomy & Physiology Student Workbook   Page 100

Please choose your answers from the box below

Abdomen	Either Side of Spine	From Iliac Crest to Top of Femur
Scapula to Humerus	Upper Back	Sides of Ribcage
Top of Scapula	Underneath Internal Obliques	Below External Obliques
Sides of Waist	Chest	Top of Scapula
Buttock	Underneath Gluteus Maximus	Between Spine & Scapula
Shoulder	From Lower Thoracic Vertebrae	Scapula
Scapula to Humerus	Back to Top of Femur	

Exercise 8

In the table below, match the muscles of the leg with their corresponding actions. Choose from the answers in the box at the end of this exercise. Please note, some actions may be repeated.

1.	Flexion & lateral rotation of the femur	
2.	Dorsiflexion & inversion of the foot, extension of big toe	
3.	Extension of knee	
4.	Flexion of the knee and extension of the hip	
5.	Plantarflexion of the foot	
6.	Flexion of the hip and extension of the knee	
7.	Adduction and medial rotation of thigh, flexion of knee	
8.	Plantarflexion and eversion of the foot	

9.	Adduction of the big toe	
10.	Dorsiflexion and eversion of foot, extension of the toes	
11.	Plantarflexion of the foot	
12.	Adduction and lateral rotation of the thigh	
13.	Extension of the knee	
14.	Dorsiflexion and inversion of the foot	
15.	Flexion of the thigh	
16.	Flexion of the knee and extension of the hip	
17.	Plantarflexion and inversion of foot, flexion of toes	
18.	Adduction and lateral rotation of the thigh	
19.	Extension of the knee	
20.	Dorsiflexion and eversion of the foot	
21.	Flexion of the knee & hip, lateral rotation of thigh	
22.	Plantarflexion and inversion of the foot	

23.	Flexion of the knee and extension of the hip	
24.	Plantarflexion and inversion of the foot, flexion of big toe	
25.	Extension of the knee	
26.	Plantarflexion of the foot	

Please choose your answers from the box below

Vastus Lateralis	Adductor Brevis	Extensor Digitorum Longus
Psoas	Semimembranosus	Adductor Longus
Adductor Magnus	Gracilis	Tibialis Anterior
Peroneus Brevis	Flexor Hallucis Longus	Semitendinosus
Extensor Hallucis Longus	Gastrocnemius	Vastus Medialis
Iliacus	Vastus Intermedius	Rectus Femoris
Flexor Digitorum Longus	Peroneus Tertius	
Soleus	Achilles Tendon	
Tibialis Posterior	Biceps Femoris	
Sartorius	Adductor Hallucis	

Exercise 9

Fill in the missing words.

1. The teres major adducts and _____ rotates the humerus (8)

2. The origin is the _____ end of the muscle (5)

3. Skeletal muscle is a type of muscle that we _____ control (11)

4. The levator labii superioris lifts the _____ lip (5)

5. The _____ is positioned underneath the gastrocnemius (6)

6. The extensor digitorum _____ extends the toes (6)

7. The splenius capitis is responsible for _____ of the head and neck (9)

8. The masseter is the main muscle of _____ (11)

9. The gastrocnemius is also known as the _____ muscle (4)

10. The _____ flex the knee and extend the hip (10)

11. Myositis describes _____ of a muscle (12)

12. _____ muscle is involuntary (6)

13. The _____ pterygoid pushes the mandible out (7)

14. The _____ is positioned in the upper back (9)

15. The coracobrachialis flexes and _____ the humerus (7)

16. The tibialis anterior is positioned on the _____front of the lower leg (7)

17. The _____ adduct the scapula (9)

18. The brachialis _____ the elbow joint (6)

19. The levator _____ oris lifts the angle of the mouth (6)

20. The _____ extend the forearm (7)

Exercise 10

In the table below, match the muscles of the torso with their corresponding actions. Choose from the answers in the box at the end of this exercise. Please note, some actions may be repeated.

1.	Lifts the shoulders	
2.	Abduction and medial rotation of the thigh	
3.	Draws the ribcage upwards	
4.	Draws shoulder downwards and forwards	
5.	Abduction of humerus	
6.	Flexion and rotation of the trunk	
7.	Raises the shoulders and rotation of the scapula	
8.	Lateral Flexion of lumbar vertebrae	
9.	Adduction and medial rotation of humerus	
10.	Extension of vertebral column	
11.	Draws scapula forwards	
12.	Supports the abdominal organs	

Anatomy & Physiology Student Workbook — Page 105

13.	Extension of thigh at hip and lateral rotation of thigh	
14.	Lateral rotation of humerus	
15.	Adduction and medial rotation of the arm	
16.	Draws ribcage downwards	
17.	Lateral rotation of humerus	
18.	Extension, adduction and medial rotation of the arm	
19.	Flexes the vertebral column	
20.	Adduction of scapula	
21.	Medial rotation of the humerus	
22.	Flexion and rotation of the trunk	

Please choose your answers from the box below

Transverse Abdominis	Trapezius	External Intercostals
Rhomboids	Teres Minor	Subscapularis
Levator Scapulae	Rectus Abdominis	External Oblique
Supraspinatus	Internal Intercostals	Serratus Anterior
Pectoralis Major	Quadratus Lumborum	Gluteus Medius
Internal Oblique	Latissimus Dorsi	Pectoralis Minor
Gluteus Maximus	Infraspinatus	
Erector Spinae	Teres Major	

Exercise 11

In the table below, match the muscles of the arm and hand with their corresponding actions. Choose from the answers in the box at the end of this exercise. Please note, some actions may be repeated.

1.	Abduction of arm		14.	Draws arm backwards	
2.	Flexion of fingers		15.	Flexion and supination of forearm	
3.	Extension of wrist		16.	Extension of thumb	
4.	Flexion of little finger		17.	Flexion and abduction of thumb	
5.	Thumb flexion		18.	Extension of fingers	
6.	Pronation and flexion of the forearm		19.	Flexes forearm at the elbow	
7.	Draws arm forwards		20.	Extension of wrist	
8.	Flexes distal phalanges		21.	Flexion of middle phalanges	
9.	Flexion of wrist		22.	Flexion of hand	
10.	Flexion of forearm		23.	Supination of forearm	

Anatomy & Physiology Student Workbook

11.	Abduction and flexion of little finger		24.	Flexion of wrist	
12.	Flexion and adduction of the arm		25.	Extension of forearm	
13.	Abduction of thumb				

Please choose your answers from the box below

Flexor Carpi Radialis	Brachialis	Flexor Digiti Minimi
Triceps	Flexor Carpi Digitorum	Extensor Carpi Ulnaris
Middle Deltoid	Opponens Pollicis	Biceps
Coracobrachialis	Palmaris Longus	Abductor Pollicis Brevis
Anterior Deltoid	Pronator Teres	Flexor Digitorum Profundas
Flexor Carpi Ulnaris	Posterior Deltoid	Extensor Pollicis Longus
Brachioradialis	Supinator Radii Brevis	Flexor Digitorum Superficialis
Extensor Carpi Radialis	Flexor Pollicis Brevis	
Abductor Digiti Minimi	Extensor Digitorum	

Anatomy & Physiology Student Workbook

Exercise 12

Multiple choice questions, please choose one answer from the 4 choices provided in each box.

1. What muscle creates the horizontal lines between the eyebrows when drawing them together? a) Procerus b) Frontalis c) Nasalis d) Levator labii superioris Answer	2. Movement of a body part in an upwards direction is known as; a) Elevation b) Protraction c) Reduction d) Retraction Answer
3. Which one of the following is not a muscle of the hypothenar eminence? a) Abductor digiti minimi b) Opponens digiti minimi c) Abductor pollicis brevis d) Flexor digiti minimi Answer	4. What is the action of the brachioradialis? a) Flexes the wrist b) Flexes the forearm at the elbow c) Flexes the phalanges d) Extension of the wrist Answer
5. What muscle everts and plantarflexes the foot? a) Tibialis posterior b) Peroneus longus c) Tibialis anterior d) Gastrocnemius Answer	6. What muscle of the face closes the mouth? a) Corrugator b) Orbicularis oculi c) Orbicularis oris d) Procerus Answer
7. What muscle laterally rotates the thigh? a) Sartorius b) Rectus femoris c) Soleus d) Gracilis Answer	8. Circumduction describes; a) Movement in a posterior direction b) Movement in an anterior direction c) Movement in a medial direction d) Movement in a circular direction Answer

9. Which one of the following is a rotator cuff muscle? a) Levator scapula b) Trapezius c) Rhomboids d) Supraspinatus Answer	**10. What muscle is responsible for straightening the arm?** a) Triceps b) Deltoid c) Brachialis d) Biceps Answer
11. The pectoralis major is positioned in the; a) Chest b) Shoulder c) Abdominal cavity d) Leg Answer	**12. What muscle is responsible for bending the lumbar vertebrae to the side?** a) Gluteus minimus b) Rectus abdominis c) Gluteus maximus d) Quadratus lumborum Answer
13. What type of muscle tissue consists of myofibrils? a) Cardiac b) Skeletal c) Smooth d) Involuntary Answer	**14. If you had tight, short pectoralis muscles what postural deformity might you suffer from?** a) Lordosis b) Kyphosis c) Scoliosis d) Atony Answer
15. What is the action of the splenius capitis? a) Extension of the neck b) Flexion of the neck c) Rotation of the head from side to side d) Extension of the trunk Answer	**16. Lateral epicondylitis is another term for;** a) Frozen shoulder b) Muscle inflammation c) Golfer's elbow d) Tennis elbow Answer

Anatomy & Physiology Student Workbook

17. What muscle is positioned at the back of the head? a) Frontalis b) Temporalis c) Occipitalis d) Corrugator Answer	18. What disorder of the muscular system is caused by constant repetition of certain movements? a) Fibrositis b) Muscle spasm c) Muscle strain d) RSI Answer
19. What muscle is used when smiling? a) Nasalis b) Zygomaticus c) Lateral pterygoid d) Mentalis Answer	20. What muscle is positioned beneath the internal obliques? a) Rectus abdominis b) Transverse abdominis c) External obliques d) Serratus anterior Answer
21. What type of tissue are tendons made up of? a) Elastic b) Adipose c) Fibrous d) Areolar Answer	22. What muscle raises the lower jaw? a) Masseter b) Mentalis c) Risorius d) Orbicularis oculi Answer
23. Which one of the following is not a muscle of the thenar eminence? a) Abductor pollicis brevis b) Opponens digiti minimi c) Opponens pollicis d) Flexor pollicis brevis Answer	24. What is the action of the teres major? a) Lateral rotation of the humerus b) Abduction of the humerus c) Adduction of the humerus d) Elevation of the shoulders Answer

25. What muscle flexes the trunk?
a) Transverse abdominis
b) Rectus abdominis
c) Erector spinae
d) Latissimus dorsi

Answer

26. Which one of the following is not a function of the muscular system?
a) Movement
b) Production of heat
c) Maintenance of posture
d) Storage

Answer

27. What protein strands are found within myofibrils?
a) Glycogen and lactic acid
b) Rennin and lipase
c) Actin and myosin
d) Glucose and myosin

Answer

28. What is the action of the pectoralis major?
a) Adducts and medially rotates the arm
b) Abducts the humerus
c) Flexes the forearm at the elbow
d) Elevation of the scapula

Answer

29. What muscle is positioned at the back of the humerus?
a) Brachialis
b) Coracobrachialis
c) Triceps
d) Pronator teres

Answer

30. What muscle is used when winking?
a) Orbicularis oculi
b) Corrugator
c) Orbicularis oris
d) Temporalis

Answer

31. What muscle separates the thoracic cavity from the abdominal cavity?
a) Rectus abdominis
b) External oblique
c) Serratus anterior
d) Diaphragm

Answer

32. What muscle is positioned across the top of the back?
a) Trapezius
b) Latissimus dorsi
c) Rhomboids
d) Teres major

Answer

33. What type of muscle contraction occurs when the muscle works without moving?
a) Isometric
b) Agonist
c) Insertion
d) Isotonic

Answer

34. What is the action of the psoas muscle?
a) Lateral rotation of the hip
b) Extension of the thigh
c) Flexion of the thigh
d) Abduction of the thigh

Answer

35. What action is the flexor hallucis longus responsible for?
a) Dorsiflexion of the foot
b) Extension of the big toe
c) Flexion of the big toe
d) Flexion of the 4th and 5th toes

Answer

36. What muscle is positioned on the inside of the thigh?
a) Semitendinosus
b) Vastus medialis
c) Gracilis
d) Tibialis anterior

Answer

37. What covers a muscle?
a) Tendons
b) Fascia
c) Ligaments
d) Periosteum

Answer

38. What muscle elevates the mandible?
a) Depressor anguli oris
b) Buccinator
c) Risorius
d) Medial pterygoid

Answer

39. What group of muscles mole the little finger?
a) Extension digitorum
b) Quadriceps
c) Thenar eminence
d) Hypothenar eminence

Answer

40. What muscle is positioned between the eyebrows?
a) Orbicularis oculi
b) Masseter
c) Medial pterygoid
d) Procerus

Answer

The Muscular System

Answers

Exercise 1 (true/false):

1. False	11. True	21. False	31. True	41. False
2. True	12. True	22. False	32. True	42. True
3. True	13. True	23. False	33. False	43. False
4. False	14. True	24. False	34. False	44. True
5. True	15. False	25. False	35. True	45. True
6. False	16. False	26. True	36. False	46. False
7. False	17. True	27. True	37. True	47. True
8. False	18. False	28. True	38. True	48. False
9. True	19. True	29. True	39. False	49. True
10. False	20. True	30. False	40. False	50. False

Exercise 2 (match the muscles of the head and neck with their action):

1. Frontalis
2. Orbicularis Oculi
3. Depressor Labii Inferioris
4. Splenius Capitis
5. Nasalis
6. Orbicularis Oris
7. Medial Pterygoid
8. Levator Labii Superioris
9. Procerus
10. Sternocleidomastoid
11. Levator Anguli Oris
12. Temporalis
13. Zygomaticus
14. Lateral Pterygoid
15. Depressor Anguli Oris
16. Occipitalis
17. Buccinator
18. Platysma
19. Mentalis
20. Masseter

Exercise 3 (crossword):

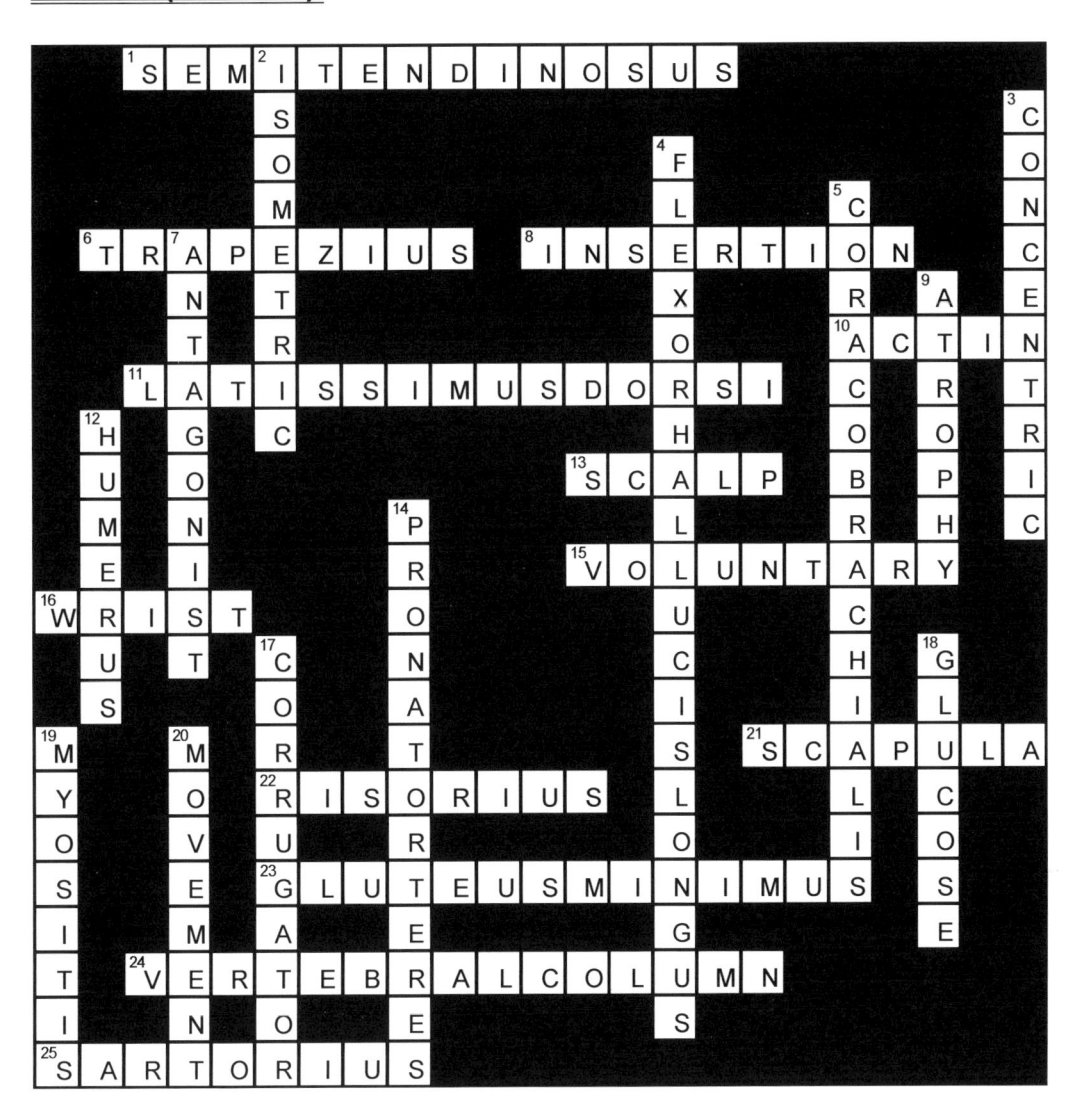

Across:
1. SEMITENDINOSUS
6. TRAPEZIUS
8. INSERTION
10. ACTIN
11. LATISSIMUSDORSI
13. SCALP
15. VOLUNTARY
16. WRIST
21. SCAPULA
22. RISORIUS
23. GLUTEUSMINIMUS
24. VERTEBRALCOLUMN
25. SARTORIUS

Exercise 4 (match the muscles of the lower limbs with their positions in the body):

1. Gracilis
2. Adductor Brevis
3. Extensor Hallucis Longus
4. Soleus
5. Biceps Femoris
6. Vastus Lateralis
7. Flexor Digitorum Longus
8. Semimembranosus
9. Vastus Intermedius
10. Peroneus Longus
11. Tibialis Anterior
12. Rectus Femoris
13. Flexor Hallucis Longus
14. Sartorius
15. Extensor Digitorum Longus
16. Semitendinosus
17. Gastrocnemius
18. Abductor Hallucis
19. Peroneus Tertius
20. Tibialis Posterior

Anatomy & Physiology Student Workbook

Exercise 5 (match the muscles of the arm and hand with their positions in the body):

1. Coracobrachialis
2. Extensor Carpi Ulnaris
3. Pronator Teres
4. Thenar Eminence
5. Triceps
6. Flexor Carpi Radialis
7. Biceps
8. Extensor Carpi Radialis
9. Flexor Carpi Ulnaris
10. Extensor Carpi Digitorum
11. Anconeus
12. Flexor Carpi Superficialis

Exercise 6 (word search):

1. Medially
2. Flexor Carpi Digitorum
3. Plantarflexion
4. Trapezius
5. Serratus Anterior
6. Mentalis
7. Supraspinatus
8. Belly
9. Zygomaticus
10. Striated
11. Triceps
12. Tibialis Anterior
13. Upper Lip
14. Pectoralis Major
15. Rhomboids
16. Quadriceps
17. Orbicularis Oculi
18. Deltoid
19. Lactic Acid
20. Involuntary
21. Forearm
22. Sartorius
23. Agonist
24. Tendon
25. Erector Spinae

Exercise 7 (match muscles of the torso with their positions in the body):

1. Either Side of Spine
2. Chest
3. Back
4. Abdomen
5. From Lower Thoracic Vertebrae to Top of Femur
6. Buttock
7. Top of Scapula
8. Sides of Ribcage
9. Between Spine & Scapula
10. Scapula to Humerus
11. Below External Obliques
12. Scapula
13. Upper Back
14. Scapula to Humerus
15. Shoulder
16. Sides of Waist
17. From Iliac Crest to Top of Femur
18. Underneath Gluteus Maximus
19. Underneath Internal Obliques
20. Top of Scapula

Anatomy & Physiology Student Workbook

Exercise 8 (match muscles of the leg with their corresponding actions):
1. Iliacus
2. Extensor Hallucis Longus
3. Vastus Intermedius/Lateralis/Medialis
4. Semimembranosus/Semitendinosus/Biceps Femoris
5. Achilles Tendon/Gastrocnemius/Soleus
6. Rectus Femoris
7. Gracilis
8. Peroneus Brevis
9. Adductor Hallucis
10. Extensor Digitorum Longus
11. Soleus/Gastrocnemius/Achilles Tendon
12. Adductor Magnus/ Adductor Longus/Adductor Brevis
13. Vastus Lateralis/Intermedius/Medialis
14. Tibialis Anterior
15. Psoas
16. Semitendinosus/Semimembranosus/Biceps Femoris
17. Flexor Digitorum Longus
18. Adductor Longus/Brevis/Magnus
19. Vastus Medialis/Lateralis/Intermedius
20. Peroneus Tertius
21. Sartorius
22. Tibialis Posterior
23. Biceps Femoris/Semimembranosus/Semitendinosus
24. Flexor Hallucis Longus
25. Vastus Medialis/Lateralis/Intermedius
26. Gastrocnemius/Soleus/Achilles Tendon

Exercise 9 (fill in the missing words):
1. Medially
2. Fixed
3. Consciously
4. Upper
5. Soleus
6. Longus
7. Extension
8. Mastication
9. Calf
10. Hamstrings
11. Inflammation
12. Smooth
13. Lateral
14. Trapezius
15. Adducts
16. Lateral
17. Rhomboids
18. Flexes
19. Anguli
20. Triceps

Exercise 10 (match the muscles of the torso with their corresponding actions):

1. Levator Scapulae
2. Gluteus Medius
3. External Intercostals
4. Pectoralis Minor
5. Supraspinatus
6. External Oblique/Internal Oblique
7. Trapezius
8. Quadratus Lumborum
9. Teres Major
10. Erector Spinae
11. Serratus Anterior
12. Transverse Abdominis
13. Gluteus Maximus
14. Infraspinatus
15. Pectoralis Major
16. Internal Intercostals
17. Teres Minor
18. Latissimus Dorsi
19. Rectus Abdominis
20. Rhomboids
21. Subscapularis
22. Internal Oblique/External Oblique

Exercise 11 (match the muscles of the arm and hand with their corresponding actions):

1. Middle Deltoid
2. Flexor Carpi Digitorum
3. Extensor Carpi Radialis
4. Flexor Digiti Minimi
5. Flexor Pollicis Brevis
6. Pronator Teres
7. Anterior Deltoid
8. Flexor Digitorum Profundas
9. Flexor Carpi Radialis
10. Brachialis
11. Abductor Digiti Minimi
12. Coracobrachialis
13. Abductor Pollicis Brevis
14. Posterior Deltoid
15. Biceps
16. Extensor Pollicis Longus
17. Opponens Pollicis
18. Extensor Digitorum
19. Brachioradialis
20. Extensor Carpi Ulnaris
21. Flexor Digitorum Superficialis
22. Palmaris Longus
23. Supinator Radii Brevis
24. Flexor Carpi Ulnaris
25. Triceps

Exercise 12 (multiple choice questions):

1	A	9	D	17	C	25	B	33	A
2	A	10	A	18	D	26	D	34	C
3	C	11	A	19	B	27	C	35	C
4	B	12	D	20	B	28	A	36	C
5	B	13	B	21	C	29	C	37	B
6	C	14	B	22	A	30	A	38	D
7	A	15	A	23	B	31	D	39	D
8	D	16	D	24	C	32	A	40	D

Chapter 5 | The Cardiovascular System

Revision Puzzles & Questions

Exercise 1

The following grid lists statements on the left that are either true or false. Please choose your answer on the right. All answers are provided at the end of the chapter.

1.	Granulocytes and thrombocytes make up leucocytes	True ☐ False ☐
2.	The endocardium is the inner wall of the heart	True ☐ False ☐
3.	The pulmonary vein carries oxygenated blood from the lungs to the heart	True ☐ False ☐
4.	The carotid veins are the main veins of the head and neck	True ☐ False ☐
5.	Systolic pressure occurs when the heart is contracting	True ☐ False ☐
6.	Bradycardia occurs when the pulse rate beats over 100 times per minute	True ☐ False ☐
7.	The pulmonary vein returns blood from the lungs to the right atrium	True ☐ False ☐

Anatomy & Physiology Student Workbook

8.	Plasma proteins include globulin, fibrinogen and haemoglobin	True ☐ False ☐
9.	Capillaries are the smallest blood vessels	True ☐ False ☐
10.	The bicuspid valve is located between the right atrium and the right ventricle	True ☐ False ☐
11.	Plasma makes up 55% of the blood's composition	True ☐ False ☐
12.	The right and left sides of the heart are divided by a muscular wall called the septum	True ☐ False ☐
13.	Deoxygenated blood enters the left atrium of the heart by the pulmonary veins	True ☐ False ☐
14.	Red blood cells are known as erythrocytes	True ☐ False ☐
15.	The pericardium is the middle layer of the heart wall	True ☐ False ☐
16.	Hypertension is another name for low blood pressure	True ☐ False ☐
17.	Type O blood is the universal donor	True ☐ False ☐

18.	The cephalic vein can be found in the arm	True ☐ False ☐
19.	Deoxygenated blood passes through the bicuspid valve into the right ventricle	True ☐ False ☐
20.	Arteries carry oxygenated blood to the lungs with the exception of the pulmonary artery	True ☐ False ☐
21.	Thrombocytes are known as platelets	True ☐ False ☐
22.	The average pulse rate of an adult is between 70 and 90 beats per minute	True ☐ False ☐
23.	The pulmonary vein branches into the right and left pulmonary veins and takes deoxygenated blood to both lungs	True ☐ False ☐
24.	Hepatitis affects the pancreas	True ☐ False ☐
25.	The aorta is the largest artery of the heart	True ☐ False ☐
26.	Monocytes produce antibodies	True ☐ False ☐
27.	Thrombin converts fibrinogen into fibrin	True ☐ False ☐

28.	Oxygenated blood is returned to the left atrium of the heart via the pulmonary veins	True ☐ False ☐
29.	Blood within the veins is carried under high pressure	True ☐ False ☐
30.	Blood pressure is recorded by a sphygmomanometer	True ☐ False ☐
31.	Vitamin B12 is required for a blood clot to form	True ☐ False ☐
32.	Leucocytes transport oxygen to the body's cells	True ☐ False ☐
33.	The upper chambers of the heart are called atria	True ☐ False ☐
34.	Arteries eventually join up to form small veins called venules	True ☐ False ☐
35.	The aorta leaves the left ventricle	True ☐ False ☐
36.	In the lungs, carbon dioxide is removed and replaced with oxygen	True ☐ False ☐
37.	Vitamin B6 is necessary for the development of erythrocytes in red bone marrow	True ☐ False ☐

38.	Lack of iron in the blood causes anaemia	True ☐ False ☐
39.	Deoxygenated blood enters the right atrium via the inferior and superior vena cava	True ☐ False ☐
40.	Anyone with type B blood can receive blood from all blood groups	True ☐ False ☐

Exercise 2

In the following table, state whether the characteristics/definitions below fall under the category of <u>Arteries, Veins, Capillaries, Venules or Arterioles</u>. All answers are at the end of the chapter.

1.	Small lumen		8.	Smaller arteries	
2.	Smallest blood vessels		9.	Thick elastic, muscular walls	
3.	Unites capillaries and veins		10.	Carry blood under low pressure	
4.	Carry blood towards the heart		11.	Valves are present to prevent backflow of blood	
5.	Small veins		12.	Large lumen	
6.	Receive blood from arterioles		13.	Carry blood away from heart	
7.	Carry blood under high pressure		14.	Nutrients and gas pass through	

Exercise 3

Complete the following crossword on The Cardiovascular System by answering the clues below.

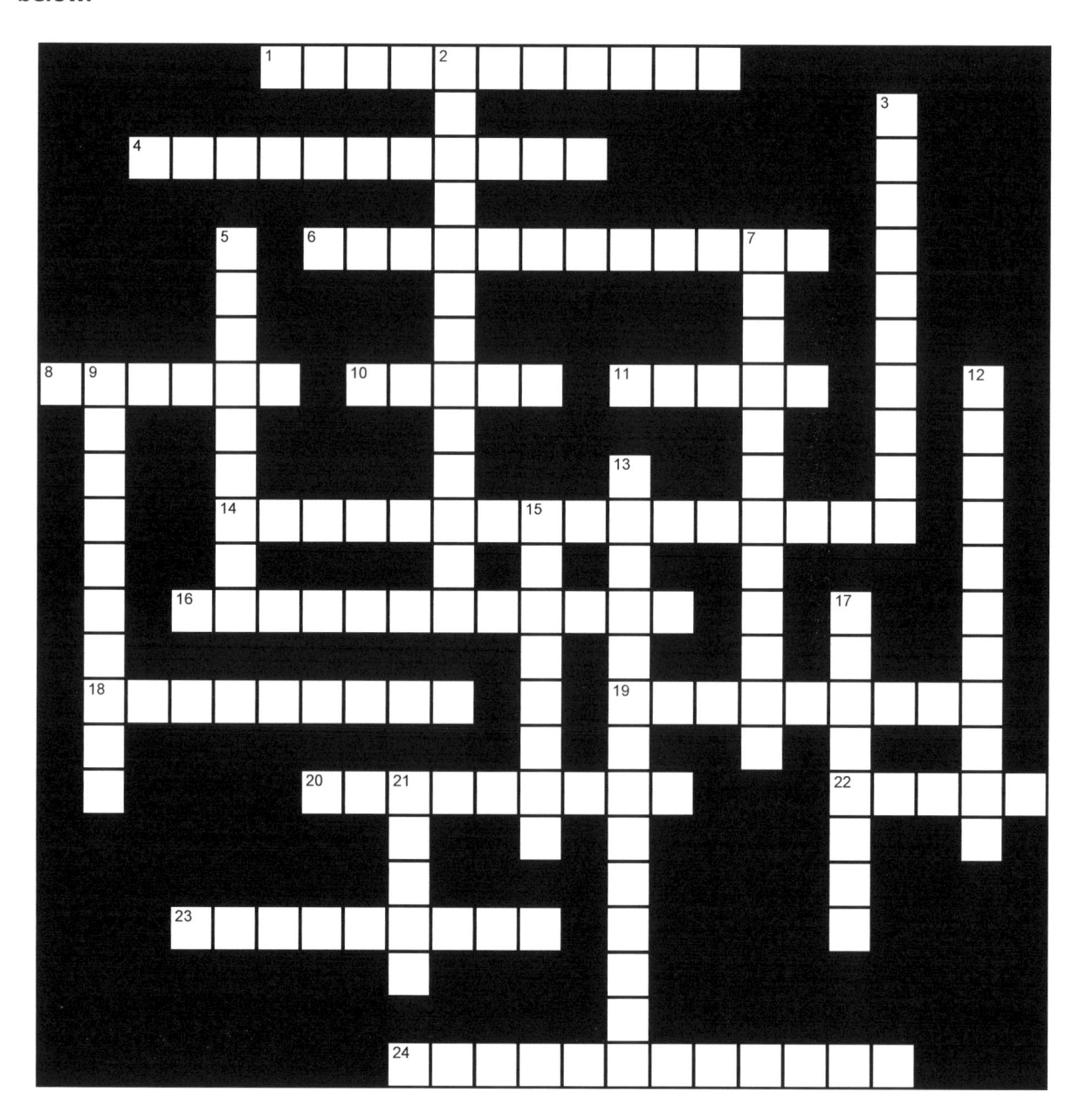

Across
1. What is the outer layer of the heart called? (11)
4. What chamber of the heart receives deoxygenated blood from the superior and inferior vena cava? (11)
6. What are platelets also known as? (12)
8. A slightly thick, clear, pale yellow fluid (6)
10. What blood vessels carry deoxygenated blood from the heart (5)

Anatomy & Physiology Student Workbook

11. Through which artery does blood leave the heart to be transported around the body? (5)
14. A disease of the cardiovascular system causes the walls of vessels to lose elasticity (16)
16. What is the term used to describe high blood pressure? (12)
18. Valve preventing the backflow of oxygenated blood from the right ventricle to right atria (9)
19. At what point in the right atrium does the heartbeat begin? (9)
20. What is inflammation of a vein known as? (9)
22. What type of blood is known as the universal donor? (5)
23. What is cancer of the blood called? (9)
24. What type of blood travels from the heart to the lungs in the pulmonary artery? (12)

Down
2. What is removed from the blood when it arrives in the lungs? (13)
3. What are the lower chambers of the heart called? (10)
5. What type of circulation carries blood from the heart to the lungs? (9)
7. What type of blood cells are found in red bone marrow? (12)
9. What type of cells protect the body against infection? (10)
12. What are the smallest blood vessels? (11)
13. What is septicaemia? (14)
15. What type of circulation is the circulation of blood from the heart to the upper & lower body? (8)
17. What is the heart's resting period called? (8)
21. What organ does hepatitis affect? (5)

Exercise 4

Circulation of the blood throughout the body goes through 9 stages. Please match the stages in the table below. Stage 1 has been completed for you.

1.	**Deoxygenated blood from the body flows through the superior and inferior vena cava, emptying into the right atrium**	Stage 1
2.	In the lungs, carbon dioxide is removed from the lungs and replaced with oxygen	
3.	Blood is then passed through the pulmonary valve into the pulmonary artery	
4.	Oxygenated blood leaves the left ventricle and passes into the aorta through the aortic valve	
5.	Deoxygenated blood leaves the right atrium through the tricuspid valve into the right ventricle	
6.	Oxygenated blood is returned from the lungs to the left atrium of the heart via the pulmonary veins	
7.	The aorta transports oxygenated blood around the body supplying oxygen and nutrients to the cells	
8.	The pulmonary artery divides into the left and right branches and carries the blood into both sides of the lungs	
9.	Oxygenated blood leaves the left atrium and passes into the left ventricle via the bicuspid	

Exercise 5

Please answer the questions below and find the answers in the word search puzzle.

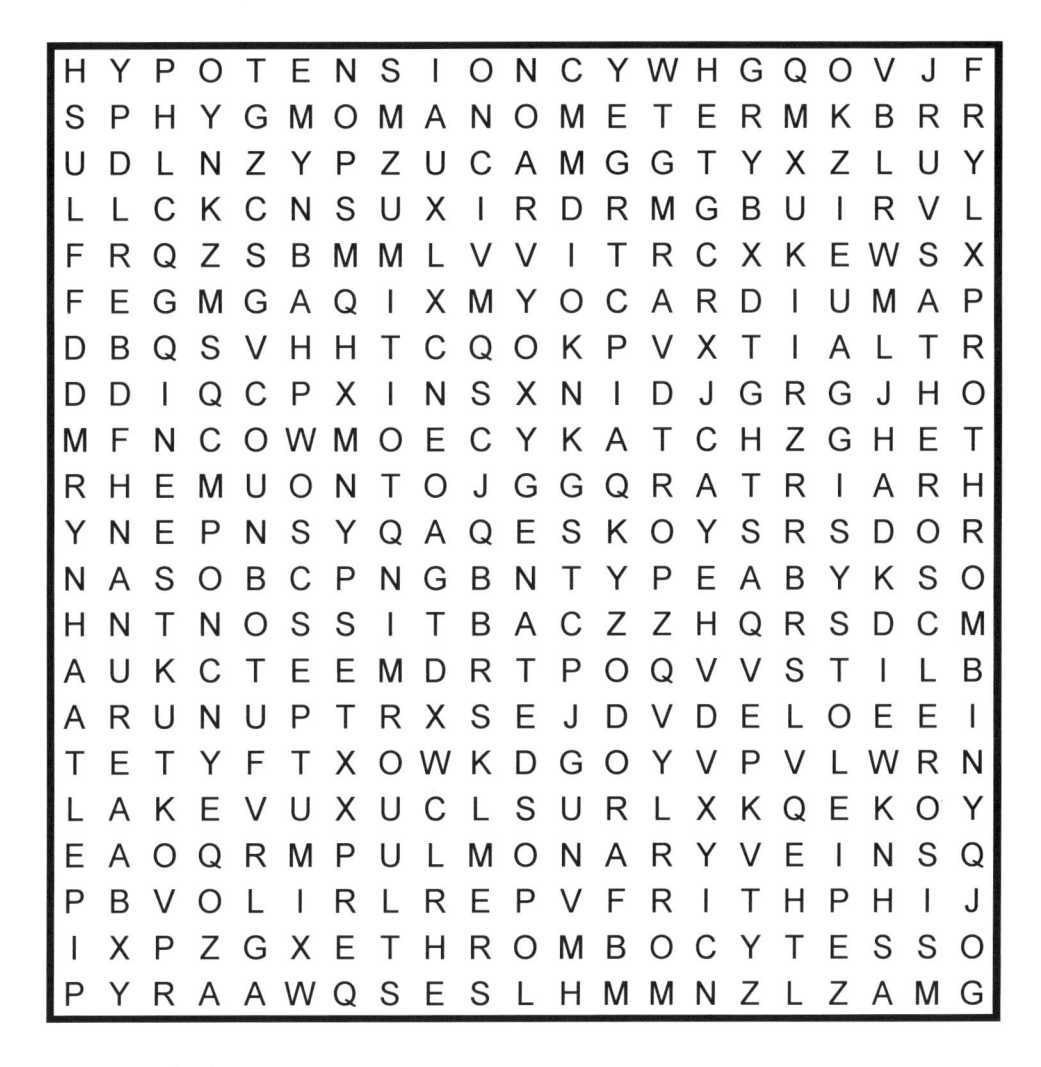

```
H Y P O T E N S I O N C Y W H G Q O V J F
S P H Y G M O M A N O M E T E R M K B R R
U D L N Z Y P Z U C A M G G T Y X Z L U Y
L L C K C N S U X I R D R M G B U I R V L
F R Q Z S B M M L V V I T R C X K E W S X
F E G M G A Q I X M Y O C A R D I U M A P
D B Q S V H H T C Q O K P V X T I A L T R
D D I Q C P X I N S X N I D J G R G J H O
M F N C O W M O E C Y K A T C H Z G H E T
R H E M U O N T O J G G Q R A T R I A R H
Y N E P N S Y Q A Q E S K O Y S R S D O R
N A S O B C P N G B N T Y P E A B Y K S O
H N T N O S S I T B A C Z Z H Q R S D C M
A U K C T E E M D R T P O Q V V S T I L B
A R U N U P T R X S E J D V D E L O E E I
T E T Y F T X O W K D G O Y V P V L W R N
L A K E V U X U C L S U R L X K Q E K O Y
E A O Q R M P U L M O N A R Y V E I N S Q
P B V O L I R L R E P V F R I T H P H I J
I X P Z G X E T H R O M B O C Y T E S S O
P Y R A A W Q S E S L H M M N Z L Z A M G
```

1. A plasma protein (11)
2. White blood cells (10)
3. What cells are responsible for blood clotting? (12)
4. What are the upper chambers of the heart called? (5)
5. What separates the left and right sides of the heart? (6)
6. What is the middle layer of the heart called? (10)
7. What part of the nervous system controls the actions of the heart? (9)
8. Through which vessel does deoxygenated blood travel from the heart to the lungs? (15)
9. How is the direction of blood flow controlled? (6)
10. Valve controlling backflow of deoxygenated blood from the left ventricle to left atrium (8)
11. What type of blood is received by the left atrium? (10)
12. What blood vessels carry oxygenated blood from the heart? (8)
13. What is the term used to describe low blood pressure? (11)

14. What disease of the cardiovascular system describes a build up of cholesterol along the lining of the walls of the arteries? (15)
15. What is the blood's inability to clot known as? (11)
16. What is the heart's moving period called? (7)
17. What blood vessel does oxygenated blood travel from the lungs to the heart? (13)
18. What blood group can receive blood from any blood group? (6)
19. What is used to measure blood pressure? (16)

Exercise 6

Fill in the missing words

1. Erythrocytes carry oxygen to cells and carry _____ _____ away from the cells (6,7)

2. Oxygenated blood leaves the left atrium and passes into the left ventricle via the _____ valve (8)

3. Arteries carry blood _____ from the heart (4)

4. _____ blood enters the right atrium via the superior and inferior vena cava (12)

5. The endocardium is the _____ layer of the heart (5)

6. The _____ carotid artery supplies oxygenated blood to the brain (8)

7. Blood pressure is measured in millimetres of _____ (7)

8. The _____ valve is found between the right atrium and right ventricle (9)

9. Capillaries are the _____ vessels (8)

10. The _____ _____ carries deoxygenated blood to the lungs (9,6)

11. _____ circulation involves the transport of blood from the heart to the lungs (9)

12. The veins have _____ walls (4)

13. The _____ distributes oxygenated blood throughout the body (5)

14. Antibodies help to _____ the body (7)

15. The right and left side of the heart is divided by the _____ (6)

16. The rest period between heart contractions is known as _____ pressure (9)

17. The _____ vein is found in the leg (9)

18. Agranulocytes are divided into _____ and lymphocytes (9)

19. The pulmonary veins leave the lungs carrying _____ blood to the heart (10)

20. Blood is a type of _____ tissue (10)

Exercise 7

Multiple choice questions, please choose one answer from the 4 choices provided in each box.

1. Where is the protein, haemoglobin found? a) Erythrocytes b) Thrombocytes c) Monocytes d) Leucocytes Answer	2. What valve is found between the right atrium and the right ventricle? a) Mitral b) Pulmonary c) Bicuspid d) Tricuspid Answer
3. What percentage of plasma is found in the blood? a) 40% b) 92% c) 55% d) 5% Answer	4. The heart rate of an average healthy person should be; a) 75 – 85 beats per minute b) 60 – 70 beats per minute c) 80 – 90 beats per minute d) 55 – 60 beats per minute Answer
5. Which one of the following is not a vein of the body? a) Jugular b) Saphenous c) Renal d) Basilic Answer	6. Phlebitis describes; a) Inflammation of the heart muscle b) Inflammation of the wall of the artery c) Inflammation of the wall of the vein d) Blood clot in the heart Answer

7. Which one of the following is needed for the formation of a blood clot?
a) Resin
b) Elastin
c) Fibrin
d) Vitamin A

Answer

8. What substance is removed from the blood when it reaches the lungs?
a) Haemoglobin
b) Carbon dioxide
c) Oxygen
d) Carbon monoxide

Answer

9. What category of tissue does blood fall under?
a) Connective
b) Cardiac
c) Muscular
d) Nervous

Answer

10. Ventricles are;
a) The lower chambers of the heart
b) The layers of the heart's wall
c) The valves preventing the backflow of blood
d) The upper chambers of the heart

Answer

11. What is the thickest layer of the heart?
a) Pericardium
b) Septum
c) Myocardium
d) Endocardium

Answer

12. Inflammation of the liver is known as;
a) Phlebitis
b) Hepatitis
c) Septicaemia
d) Haemophilia

Answer

13. The subclavian artery supplies what part of the body?
a) Neck
b) Thoracic wall
c) Right leg
d) Abdominal wall

Answer

14. What blood vessel leaves the heart carrying deoxygenated blood to the lungs?
a) Pulmonary artery
b) Pulmonary vein
c) Inferior vena cava
d) Aorta

Answer

15. Systemic circulation describes;
a) Circulation of deoxygenated blood from the heart to the lungs
b) Circulation of deoxygenated blood from the left ventricle to the lungs via the pulmonary artery
c) Circulation of oxygenated blood from the heart to the body
d) Circulation of oxygenated blood from the right ventricle of the heart through the aorta

Answer

16. What vein drains blood from the upper body?
a) Temporal vein
b) Pulmonary vein
c) Aorta
d) Superior vena cava

Answer

17. What regulates the flow of blood throughout the heart?
a) Valves
b) Ventricles
c) Veins
d) Arteries

Answer

18. What group of cells are not found in the blood?
a) Thrombocytes
b) Granulocytes
c) Osteoblasts
d) Erythrocytes

Answer

19. What is the function of capillaries?
a) To deliver blood to the arteries
b) To supply tissues and cells with nutrients
c) To transport blood from the heart
d) To carry deoxygenated blood from the veins

Answer

20. Deoxygenated blood from the body enters the;
a) Pulmonary vein
b) Superior and inferior vena cava
c) Aorta
d) Pulmonary artery

Answer

21. Which one of the following arteries supplies the arm?
a) Axillary
b) Femoral
c) Tibial
d) Innominate

Answer

22. What is the function of the aorta?
a) Carry oxygenated blood around the body
b) Carry oxygenated blood to the heart
c) Carry deoxygenated blood to the lungs
d) Carry deoxygenated blood from the lungs

Answer

23. Which one of the following is not a layer of the heart? a) Pericardium b) Bicuspid c) Myocardium d) Endocardium Answer	24. What group of blood cells protect the body against infection? a) Fibroblasts b) Thrombocytes c) Erythrocytes d) Leucocytes Answer
25. Hypotension describes; a) High blood pressure b) Systolic blood pressure c) Low blood pressure d) Cardiac output Answer	26. What blood type can be given to any blood group? a) AB b) O c) B d) A Answer
27. What is another term used to describe the heartbeat? a) Pulse b) Blood pressure c) Pulmonary circulation d) Cardiac cycle Answer	28. What substance gives blood its red colour? a) Mitochondria b) Fibrin c) Fibrinogen d) Oxyhaemoglobin Answer
29. What blood vessels unite arterioles and venules? a) Capillaries b) Veins c) Arteries d) Pulmonary veins Answer	30. Myocardial infarction is more commonly known as; a) Angina b) Heart attack c) High blood pressure d) Phlebitis Answer

Anatomy & Physiology Student Workbook

31. The right ventricle pushes blood into the; a) Bicuspid valve b) Pulmonary vein c) Pulmonary artery d) Aorta Answer	**32. Which one of the following is not an artery of the body?** a) Carotid b) Inferior vena cava c) Iliac d) Hepatic Answer
33. What valve is found between the left atrium and the left ventricle? a) Bicuspid b) Circulatory c) Pulmonary d) Semi lunar Answer	**34. Deoxygenated blood fills the;** a) Aortic valve b) Left atrium c) Septum d) Right atrium Answer
35. Diastolic refers to; a) When the heart muscle relaxes b) When the heart muscle contracts c) When the heart muscle fills up with blood d) When the heart muscle transports blood to the lungs Answer	**36. Thrombocytes are also known as;** a) White blood cells b) Blood corpuscles c) Platelets d) Red blood cells Answer
37. What condition describes the loss of elasticity from the walls of the arteries? a) Haemophilia b) Thrombus c) Atherosclerosis d) Arteriosclerosis Answer	**38. Oxygenated blood leaves the left ventricle through;** a) Aorta b) Pulmonary vein c) Pulmonary artery d) Superior vena cava Answer

39. Myocardium describes;	40. What are the heart's lower chambers called?
a) The wall dividing the left and right sides of the heart	a) Aorta
b) The inner layer of the heart	b) Ventricles
c) The process of muscular contraction	c) Atrium
d) The middle layer of the heart	d) Vena cava
Answer _____	**Answer** _____

The Cardiovascular System

Answers

Exercise 1 (true/false):

1. False	11. True	21. True	31. False
2. True	12. True	22. False	32. False
3. True	13. False	23. False	33. True
4. False	14. True	24. False	34. False
5. True	15. False	25. True	35. True
6. False	16. False	26. False	36. True
7. False	17. True	27. True	37. False
8. False	18. True	28. True	38. True
9. True	19. False	29. False	39. True
10. False	20. True	30. True	40. False

Exercise 2 (state whether characteristics are arteries, veins, capillaries, venules or arterioles):

1. Arteries	8. Arterioles
2. Capillaries	9. Arteries
3. Venules	10. Veins
4. Veins	11. Veins
5. Venules	12. Veins
6. Capillaries	13. Arteries
7. Arteries	14. Capillaries

Exercise 3 (crossword):

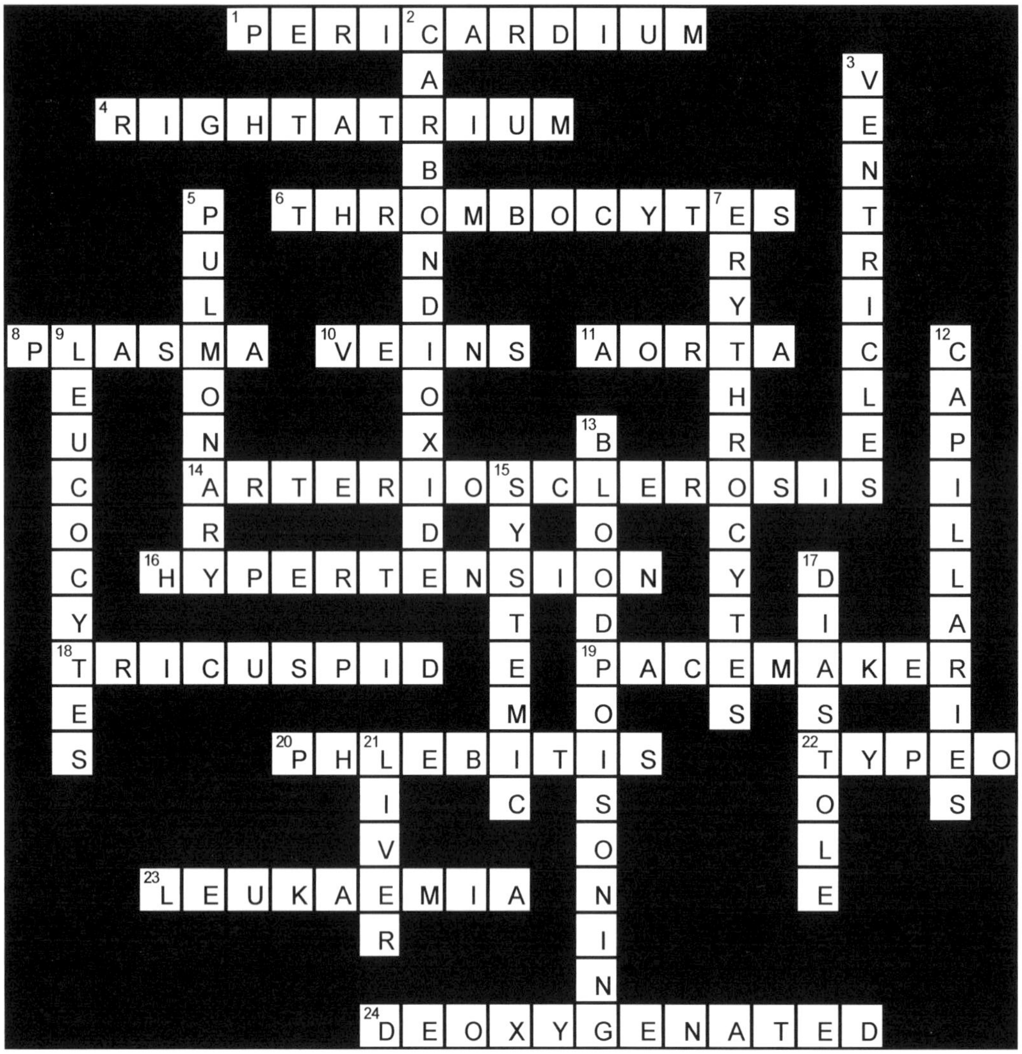

1 PERICARDIUM
2 CARBON DIOXIDE
3 VENTRICLES
4 RIGHTATRIUM
5 PULMONARY
6 THROMBOCYTES
7 ERYTHROCYTES
8 PLASMA
9 LEUCOCYTES
10 VEINS
11 AORTA
12 CAPILLARIES
13 BLOODPOISONING
14 ARTERIOSCLEROSIS
15 SYSTEMIC
16 HYPERTENSION
17 DIASTOLE
18 TRICUSPID
19 PACEMAKER
20 PHLEBITIS
21 LIVER
22 TYPEO
23 LEUKAEMIA
24 DEOXYGENATED

Exercise 4 (blood circulation occurs in 9 stages, match each stage):

1. Stage 1
2. Stage 5
3. Stage 3
4. Stage 8
5. Stage 2
6. Stage 6
7. Stage 9
8. Stage 4
9. Stage 7

Exercise 5 (word search):

1. Prothrombin
2. Leucocytes
3. Thrombocytes
4. Atria
5. Septum
6. Myocardium
7. Autonomic
8. Pulmonary Artery
9. Valves
10. Bicuspid
11. Oxygenated
12. Arteries
13. Hypotension
14. Atherosclerosis
15. Haemophilia
16. Systole
17. Pulmonary Vein
18. Type AB
19. Sphygmomanometer

Exercise 6 (fill in the missing words):

1. Carbon Dioxide
2. Bicuspid
3. Away
4. Deoxygenated
5. Inner
6. Internal
7. Mercury
8. Tricuspid
9. Smallest
10. Pulmonary Artery
11. Pulmonary
12. Thin
13. Aorta
14. Protect
15. Septum
16. Diastolic
17. Saphenous
18. Monocytes
19. Oxygenated
20. Connective

Exercise 7 (multiple choice questions):

1	A	9	A	17	A	25	C	33	A
2	D	10	A	18	C	26	B	34	D
3	C	11	C	19	B	27	D	35	A
4	B	12	B	20	B	28	D	36	C
5	C	13	B	21	A	29	A	37	D
6	C	14	A	22	A	30	B	38	A
7	C	15	C	23	B	31	C	39	D
8	B	16	D	24	C	32	B	40	B

Chapter 6 | The Lymphatic System

Revision Puzzles & Questions

Exercise 1

The following grid lists statements on the left that are either true or false. Please choose your answer on the right. All answers are provided at the end of the chapter.

1.	The lymphatic vessels have an outer layer of muscular tissue	True ☐ False ☐
2.	Lymphatic capillaries contain leucocytes and lymphocytes	True ☐ False ☐
3.	The axillary nodes are located in the underarm area	True ☐ False ☐
4.	Oedema is due to the abnormal swelling of body tissues due to the build up of excess fluid	True ☐ False ☐
5.	Lymph nodes filter the lymph	True ☐ False ☐
6.	The right lymphatic duct empties into the right subclavian vein	True ☐ False ☐
7.	Macrophages produce new antibodies to help fight infection	True ☐ False ☐

8.	Filtered lymph leaves the node by afferent vessels	True ☐ False ☐
9.	The occipital nodes are located at the base of the skull	True ☐ False ☐
10.	Lymphatic capillaries drain excess fluid towards the tissues of the body	True ☐ False ☐
11.	The spleen destroys lymphocytes	True ☐ False ☐
12.	Filtered lymph is passed into lymphatic ducts	True ☐ False ☐
13.	The popliteal nodes are located in the groin area	True ☐ False ☐
14.	Lymphatic capillaries are composed of a layer of endothelial cells	True ☐ False ☐
15.	Lymphatic vessels collect lymph from the lymphatic capillaries	True ☐ False ☐
16.	The right lymphatic duct is the largest lymphatic vessel	True ☐ False ☐
17.	Lymphatic vessels contain valves which keep the blood flowing in the right direction, preventing backflow	True ☐ False ☐

18.	Lymphatic vessels are made up of a layer of hyaline cartilage	True ☐ False ☐
19.	The thoracic duct drains lymph from the left side of the head	True ☐ False ☐
20.	The spleen is located on the right side of the abdominal cavity	True ☐ False ☐
21.	The lymph node is covered by a wall of connective tissue	True ☐ False ☐
22.	Lymphatic vessels have thin collapsible walls	True ☐ False ☐
23.	Lymphocytes produce antibodies to help fight infection	True ☐ False ☐
24.	Lymph enters the lymph nodes from the lymphatic ducts	True ☐ False ☐
25.	Cancer of the lymphatic tissue is known as Hodgkin's Disease	True ☐ False ☐
26.	The inguinal nodes are located in the elbow region	True ☐ False ☐
27.	An efferent vessel transports lymph to the lymph node	True ☐ False ☐

28.	The spleen stores blood	True ☐ False ☐
29.	Lymphatic vessels around the palm of the hand are called the plantar plexus	True ☐ False ☐
30.	The right lymphatic duct drains lymph from both lower limbs	True ☐ False ☐

Exercise 2

The transport of lymph goes through 7 main stages. Please match each stage in the table below. Stage 1 has been completed for you.

1.	Blood	Stage 1
2.	Lymphatic Vessels	
3.	Lymphatic Ducts	
4.	Venous System	
5.	Lymphatic Capillaries	
6.	Lymphatic Nodes	
7.	Subclavian Veins	

Exercise 3

Complete the following crossword on The Lymphatic System by answering the clues below.

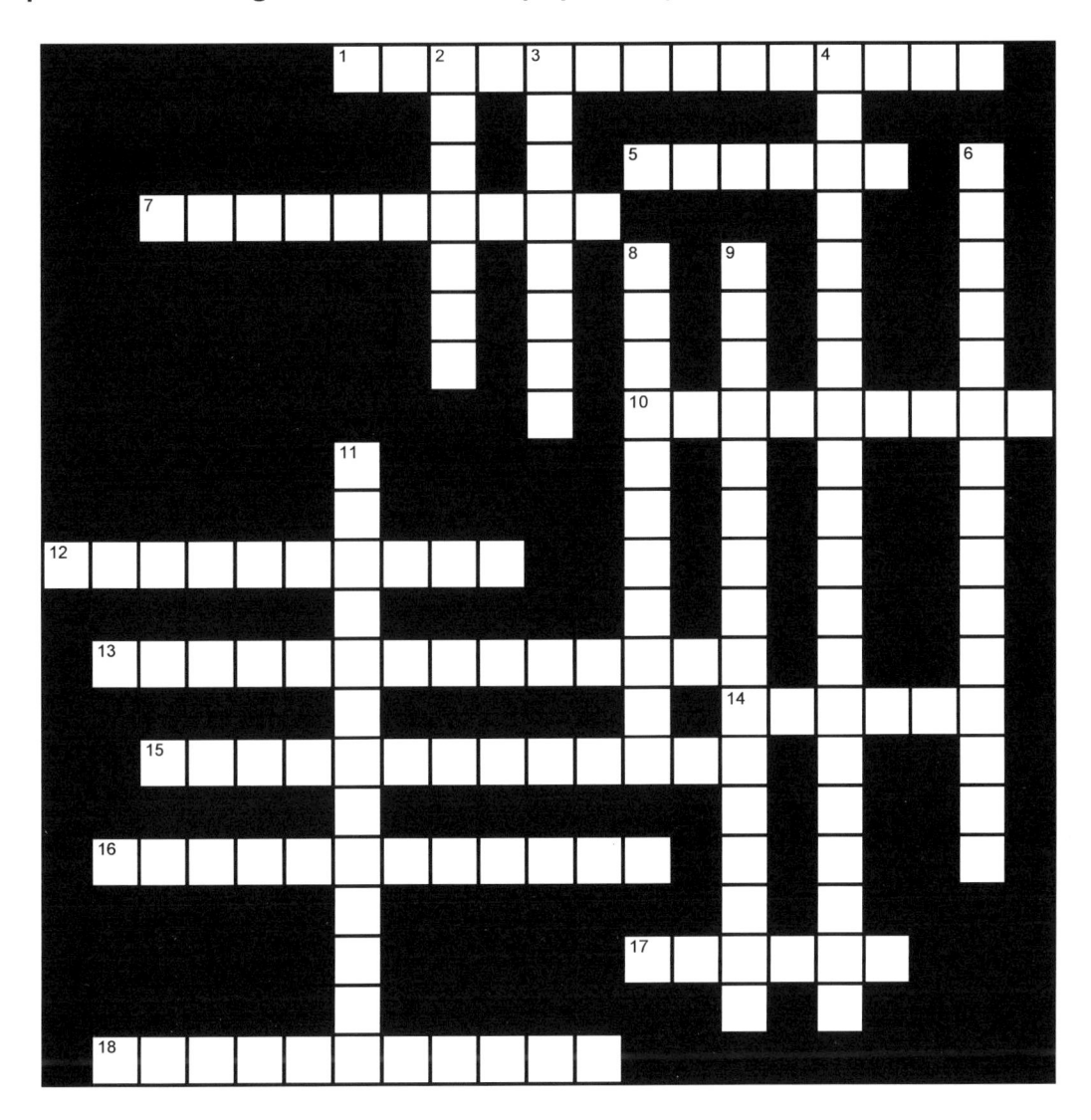

Across

1. What nodes are positioned in the elbow region? (14)
5. What disorder of the lymphatic system occurs when there is swelling in the body's tissues due to a build up of excess fluid? (6)
7. What part of the lymphatic system filters the lymph? (10)
10. What lymph node is positioned behind the knee? (9)
12. What do lymphocytes produce? (10)
13. What duct drains lymph into the right subclavian vein? (14)
14. What prevents the backflow of lymph in the lymphatic vessels? (6)
15. What type of connective tissue is the outer layer of lymphatic vessels made up of? (13)
16. What lymphatic duct drains lymph from the left side of the trunk? (12)
17. A lymphatic organ (6)

18. What does lymph transport away from the tissues? (11)

Down

2. What nodes are positioned at the angle of the jaw? (7)
3. What type of vessel transports lymph to the node? (8)
4. What carries excess fluid from the tissue spaces of the body? (20)
6. What are lymph nodes made of? (15)
8. What cells are produced in the lymph nodes? (11)
9. What part of the lymphatic system collects lymph from the lymphatic capillaries? (16)
11. What cells does the spleen destroy? (13)

Exercise 4

Fill in the missing words

1. Tissue fluid enters the _____ _____ where it becomes lymph (9, 7)

2. The thoracic duct drains lymph from the _____ arm (4)

3. The pressure inside the lymphatic capillaries is _____ than the pressure inside the blood capillaries (5)

4. The _____ nodes are located at the elbows (8)

5. The right lymphatic duct empties into the right _____ vein (10)

6. Lymphatic _____ unite to form lymphatic vessels (11)

7. Lymph has a lower level of _____ _____ than blood (6, 8)

8. Lymph passes through _____ _____ where it is filtered (5, 5)

9. The movement of lymph through the lymphatic system is known as lymphatic _____ (8)

10. The _____ nodes are located at the base of the skull (9)

11. Lymphatic vessels transport lymph _____ the heart (7)

12. The _____ system closely supports the lymphatic system (11)

13. Lymphatic vessels are made up of a layer of _____ cells (11)

14. Lymphocytes produce _____ which help to fight infection (10)

15. An efferent vessel transports _____ lymph from a lymph node (8)

Exercise 5

In the table below, match the nodes of the body with their location in the body. Choose from the answers in the box at the end of this exercise.

1.	Neck	
2.	Behind the knee	
3.	Underarms	
4.	Groin	
5.	Base of skull	
6.	Elbow	
7.	Below the mandible	
8	Thoracic cavity	
9.	Behind the ear	
10.	Pelvic cavity	

Please choose an answer from the box below

Mastoid	Popliteal
Occipital	Pelvic
Cervical	Axillary
Thoracic	Submandibular
Inguinal	Supratrochlear

Exercise 6

Please answer the questions below and find the answers in the word search puzzle.

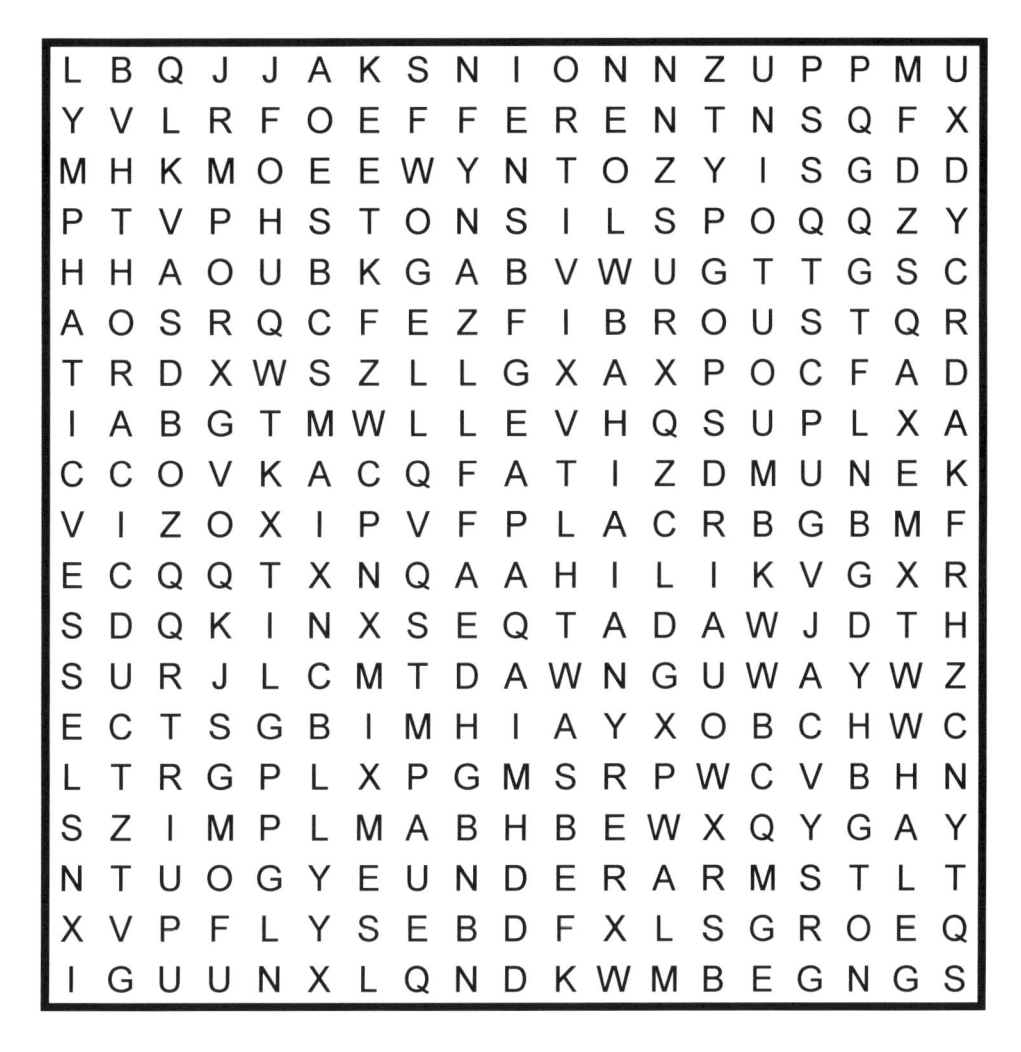

```
L B Q J J A K S N I O N N Z U P P M U
Y V L R F O E F F E R E N T N S Q F X
M H K M O E E W Y N T O Z Y I S G D D
P T V P H S T O N S I L S P O Q Q Z Y
H H A O U B K G A B V W U G T T G S C
A O S R Q C F E Z F I B R O U S T Q R
T R D X W S Z L L G X A X P O C F A D
I A B G T M W L L E V H Q S U P L X A
C C O V K A C Q F A T I Z D M U N E K
V I Z O X I P V F P L A C R B G B M F
E C Q Q T X N Q A A H I L I K V G X R
S D Q K I N X S E Q T A D A W J D T H
S U R J L C M T D A W N G U W A Y W Z
E C T S G B I M H I A Y X O B C H W C
L T R G P L X P G M S R P W C V B H N
S Z I M P L M A B H B E W X Q Y G A Y
N T U O G Y E U N D E R A R M S T L T
X V P F L Y S E B D F X L S G R O E Q
I G U U N X L Q N D K W M B E G N G S
```

1. What vessel transports filtered lymph back to the system? (8)
2. What nodes are positioned below the mandible? (13)
3. What type of tissue is found in the spleen? (7)
4. A malignant disease of the lymphatic system (15)
5. Lymphatic organs made up of lymphatic tissue (7)
6. Where are the axillary nodes positioned? (9)
7. White blood cells that destroy harmful bacteria (10)
8. What receives lymph from the lymph nodes? (14)
9. The movement of what type of muscle tissue enables lymphatic drainage? (8)
10. What nodes are found behind the knee? (9)
11. What collects lymph from the lymphatic capillaries? (16)
12. What lymphatic organ produces new lymphocytes? (6)
13. What lymphatic vessel empties into the left subclavian vein? (12)

Anatomy & Physiology Student Workbook

Exercise 7

Multiple choice questions, please choose one answer from the 4 choices provided in each box.

1. Which one of the following is not a lymphatic organ? a) Tonsils b) Spleen c) Pancreas d) Thymus gland Answer	**2. What lymphatic duct is positioned in the root of the neck?** a) Right lymphatic duct b) Subclavian duct c) Submandibular duct d) Thoracic duct Answer
3. What nodes are located in the neck? a) Cervical b) Occipital c) Submandibular d) Axillary Answer	**4. Lymphatic vessels have;** a) Thick muscular tubes b) Thin muscular tubes c) Thick collapsible walls d) Thin collapsible walls Answer
5. Which one of the following is not a function of lymph nodes? a) To filter lymph b) To destroy harmful cells c) To produce antibodies d) To produce erythrocytes Answer	**6. Which of the following drains lymph from the nose and ears?** a) Occipital b) Parotid c) Inguinal d) Popliteal Answer
7. What duct collects the most lymph? a) Subclavian duct b) Right lymphatic duct c) Right subclavian duct d) Thoracic duct Answer	**8. Which one of the following systems has a close relationship with the lymphatic system?** a) Respiratory b) Circulatory c) Nervous d) Reproductive Answer

9. What is the function of lymphatic vessels? a) To carry lymph towards the heart b) To carry lymph away from the heart c) To empty lymph into the lymphatic capillaries d) To destroy harmful waste and bacteria Answer _____	**10. What type of cells are produced by the spleen?** a) Thrombocytes b) Osteocytes c) Lymphocytes d) Erythrocytes Answer _____
11. Any obstruction in the flow of lymph is known as; a) Diabetes insipidus b) Hodgkin's disease c) Oedema d) Lymphoma Answer _____	**12. What vessels bring lymph to be filtered?** a) Plasma b) Efferent c) Blood d) Afferent Answer _____
13. What are lymph nodes made of? a) Adipose tissue b) Lymphatic tissue c) Yellow elastic cartilage d) Endothelial cells Answer _____	**14. What is the position of the spleen?** a) On the posterior wall of the abdominal cavity b) On the left of the abdominal cavity c) On the right of the abdominal cavity d) On the anterior wall of the abdominal cavity Answer _____
15. What cells produce antibodies? a) Phagocytes b) Macrophages c) Erythrocytes d) Lymphocytes Answer _____	**16. What lymphatic organ stores blood?** a) Thymus gland b) Spleen c) Tonsils d) Bladder Answer _____

17. What is the function of lymphatic capillaries?
a) To convey lymph back to the bloodstream
b) To convey excess fluid towards the tissues of the body
c) To convey excess fluid away from tissue space
d) To convey lymph towards the heart

Answer
_____

18. What group of cells are not found in the blood?
a) Thrombocytes
b) Granulocytes
c) Osteoblasts
d) Erythrocytes

Answer
_____

19. What nodes are located in the elbow region?
a) Inguinal
b) Auricular
c) Submandibular
d) Supratrochlear

Answer
_____

20. What valves prevent the backflow of lymph through lymphatic vessels?
a) Bicuspid
b) Semi lunar
c) Tricuspid
d) Mitral

Answer
_____

The Lymphatic System

Answers

Exercise 1 (true/false):

1. False	11. False	21. True
2. False	12. True	22. True
3. True	13. False	23. True
4. True	14. True	24. False
5. True	15. True	25. True
6. True	16. False	26. False
7. False	17. True	27. False
8. False	18. False	28. True
9. True	19. True	29. False
10. False	20. False	30. False

Exercise 2 (the transport of lymph goes through 7 stages, match these stages):

1. Stage 1
2. Stage 3
3. Stage 5
4. Stage 7
5. Stage 2
6. Stage 4
7. Stage 6

Exercise 3 (crossword):

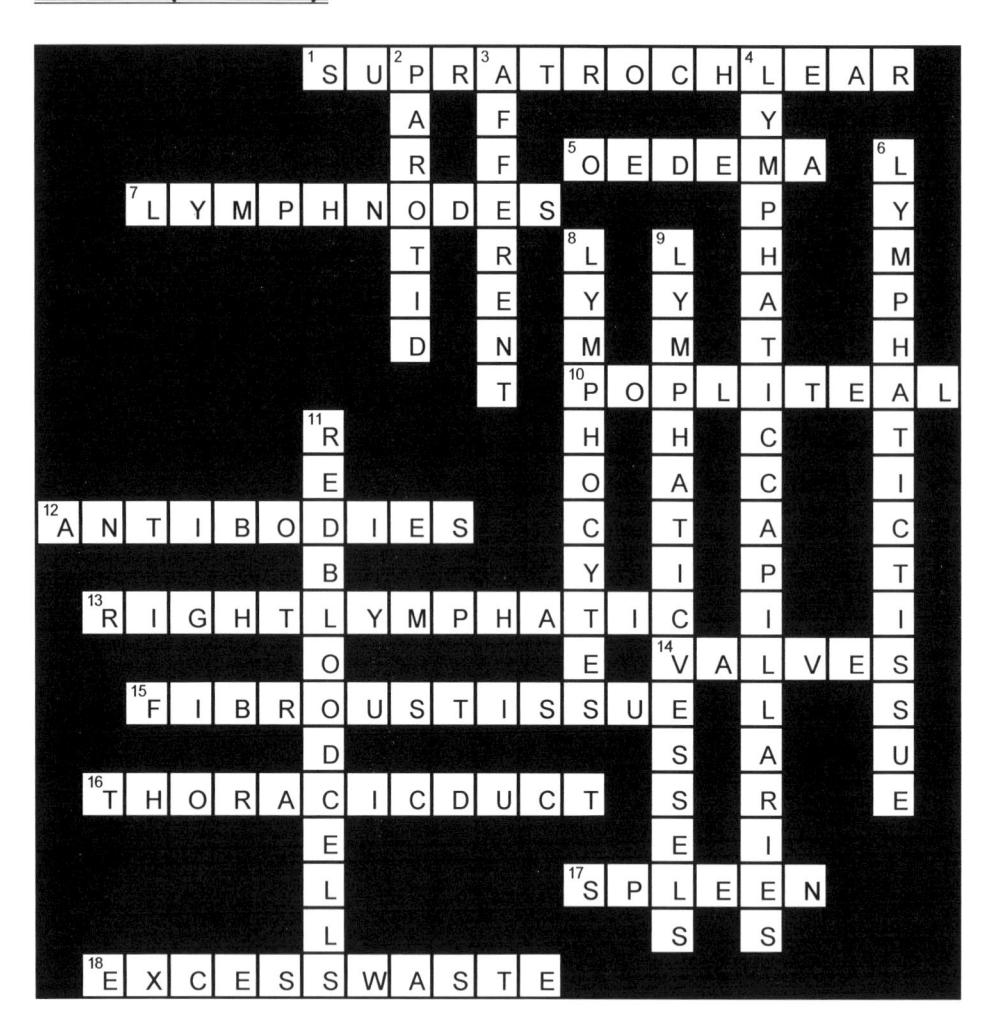

Across:
- 1. SUPRATROCHLEAR
- 5. OEDEMA
- 7. LYMPHNODES
- 10. POPLITEAL
- 12. ANTIBODIES
- 13. RIGHTLYMPHATIC
- 14. VALVES
- 15. FIBROUSTISSUE
- 16. THORACICDUCT
- 17. SPLEEN
- 18. EXCESSWASTE

Down:
- 2. UARTIDT
- 3. AFFERENT
- 4. LYMPH
- 6. LYMPH
- 8. LYMPHOCYTES
- 9. LYMPHATICAPILLARIES
- 11. REABSORBED

Exercise 4 (fill in the missing words):

1. Lymphatic Vessels
2. Left
3. Lower
4. Axillary
5. Subclavian
6. Capillaries
7. Plasma Proteins
8. Lymph Nodes
9. Drainage
10. Occipital
11. Towards
12. Circulatory
13. Endothelial
14. Antibodies
15. Filtered

Anatomy & Physiology Student Workbook

Exercise 5 (match the nodes of the body with their corresponding locations):
1. Cervical
2. Popliteal
3. Axillary
4. Inguinal
5. Occipital
6. Supratrochlear
7. Submandibular
8. Thoracic
9. Mastoid
10. Pelvic

Exercise 6 (word search):
1. Efferent
2. Submandibular
3. Fibrous
4. Hodgkin's Disease
5. Tonsils
6. Underarms
7. Phagocytes
8. Lymphatic Ducts
9. Skeletal
10. Popliteal
11. Lymphatic vessels
12. Spleen
13. Thoracic Duct

Exercise 7 (multiple choice questions):

1	C	9	A	17	C
2	A	10	C	18	C
3	A	11	C	19	D
4	D	12	D	20	B
5	D	13	B		
6	B	14	B		
7	D	15	D		
8	B	16	B		

Chapter 7 | The Endocrine System

Revision Puzzles & Questions

Exercise 1

The following grid lists statements on the left that are either true or false. Please choose your answer on the right. All answers are provided at the end of the chapter.

1.	The pituitary gland is known as the master gland of the endocrine system	True ☐ False ☐
2.	Human growth hormone is secreted by the posterior lobe of the pituitary gland	True ☐ False ☐
3.	ACTH controls the growth of the adrenal medulla	True ☐ False ☐
4.	MSH produces melanin in the surface layer of the skin	True ☐ False ☐
5.	Hyposecretion of antidiuretic hormone causes diabetes insipidus	True ☐ False ☐
6.	The adrenal glands are located underneath each kidney	True ☐ False ☐
7.	The thyroid gland is controlled by the anterior lobe of the pituitary gland	True ☐ False ☐

8.	Oestrogen stimulates the muscles of the uterus during childbirth	True ☐ False ☐
9.	FSH, ACTH & TSH are hormones secreted by the anterior lobe of the pituitary gland	True ☐ False ☐
10.	Hypersecretion of growth hormone leads to dwarfism	True ☐ False ☐
11.	The pineal gland is situated at the base of the brain	True ☐ False ☐
12.	The hormone melatonin is secreted by the pineal gland	True ☐ False ☐
13.	Hyposecretion of insulin causes hypoglycaemia	True ☐ False ☐
14.	Glucocorticoids is secreted by the adrenal cortex	True ☐ False ☐
15.	Hypersecretion of glucocorticoids causes cushing's syndrome	True ☐ False ☐
16.	Adrenaline and noradrenaline are secreted by the adrenal cortex	True ☐ False ☐
17.	The adrenal medulla supports the sympathetic nervous system	True ☐ False ☐

18.	Adrenaline increases the heart rate	True ☐ False ☐
19.	Progesterone is produced by the testes	True ☐ False ☐
20.	Hypersecretion of parathormone can lead to tetany	True ☐ False ☐
21.	Calcitonin is secreted by the thyroid glands	True ☐ False ☐
22.	Hyposecretion of antidiuretic hormone can lead to diabetes insipidus	True ☐ False ☐
23.	Hyposecretion of thyroid hormones leads to grave's disease	True ☐ False ☐
24.	Thymic factor is secreted by the thyroid glands	True ☐ False ☐
25.	The adrenal cortex secretes mineralocorticoids	True ☐ False ☐
26.	Hypersecretion of oestrogen in men causes breast growth	True ☐ False ☐
27.	Type 1 diabetes mellitus is caused when the pancreas cannot produce insulin	True ☐ False ☐

28.	Dysmenorrhoea describes the absence of menstruation	True ☐ False ☐
29.	The menstrual phase describes the beginning of menstruation	True ☐ False ☐
30.	Hyposecretion of oestrogen in females can lead to polycystic ovarian syndrome	True ☐ False ☐
31.	Menarche is a term used to describe the start of menstruation	True ☐ False ☐
32.	The pancreas is located below the stomach	True ☐ False ☐
33.	Hypersecretion of antidiuretic hormone leads to diabetes insipidus	True ☐ False ☐
34.	Hypersecretion of melatonin can lead to seasonal affective disorder (SAD)	True ☐ False ☐
35.	Hypersecretion of testosterone in women can lead to virilism	True ☐ False ☐
36.	The pituitary gland is controlled by the hypothalamus	True ☐ False ☐
37.	ICSH, FSH & LH are sex organ hormones	True ☐ False ☐

38.	Cells called the islets of langerhans are found in the adrenal cortex	True ☐ False ☐
39.	The ovaries produce oestrogen and progesterone	True ☐ False ☐
40.	When the body is at rest it produces the hormone noradrenaline	True ☐ False ☐

Exercise 2

In the table below, match the endocrine glands of the body with the corresponding hormones that they secrete. Choose from the answers in the box at the end of this exercise. Please note, some glands may be repeated.

1.	Gonadotrophins		12.	Parathormone	
2.	Melatonin		13.	Melanocyte Stimulating Hormone	
3.	Mineralocorticoids		14.	Noradrenaline	
4.	Testosterone		15.	Triodothyronine	
5.	Thyroxin		16.	Antidiuretic Hormone	
6.	Adrenaline		17.	Glucocorticoids	
7.	Human Growth Hormone		18.	Progesterone	
8.	Calcitonin		19.	Thymic Factor	
9.	Oestrogen		20.	Thyrotrophin	
10.	Insulin		21.	Oxytocin	
11.	Prolactin		22.	Adrenocorticotrophin	

Anatomy & Physiology Student Workbook

Please choose your answers from the box below

Anterior Lobe of the Pituitary Gland	Adrenal Cortex
Adrenal Cortex	Anterior Lobe of the Pituitary Gland
Pancreas	Adrenal Medulla
Anterior lobe of the Pituitary Gland	Ovaries
Testes	Posterior Lobe of the Pituitary Gland
Ovaries	Thyroid Glands
Posterior Lobe of the Pituitary Gland	Anterior Lobe of the Pituitary Gland
Thymus	Thyroid Glands
Anterior Lobe of the Pituitary Gland	Adrenal Medulla
Pineal Body	Thyroid Glands
Parathyroid Glands	Anterior Lobe of the Pituitary Gland

Exercise 3

Fill in the missing words.

1. Endocrine glands are _____ glands (8)

2. Adrenaline increases the _____ rate (9)

3. All hormones secreted by the endocrine glands pass directly into the _____ (11)

4. Gonadotrophic hormones are secreted by the _____ lobe of the pituitary gland (8)

5. The adrenal _____ secretes adrenaline and noradrenaline (7)

6. The hormone _____ is known to influence moods? (9)

7. A hormone is a _____ messenger (8)

8. Antidiuretic hormone increases _____ re absorption in the kidneys (5)

9. The _____ gland is controlled by the anterior lobe of the pituitary gland (7)

10. Tetany can be caused by the _____ of parahormone (14)

11. FSH is produced during the _____ phase of menstruation (13)

12. The testes secrete the hormone _____ (12)

13. The adrenal glands are positioned on top of each _____ (6)

14. The _____ lobe is a lobe of the pituitary gland (9)

15. The hyposecretion of thyroid hormones can lead to _____ in adults (9)

Exercise 4

Complete the following crossword on The Endocrine System by answering the clues below.

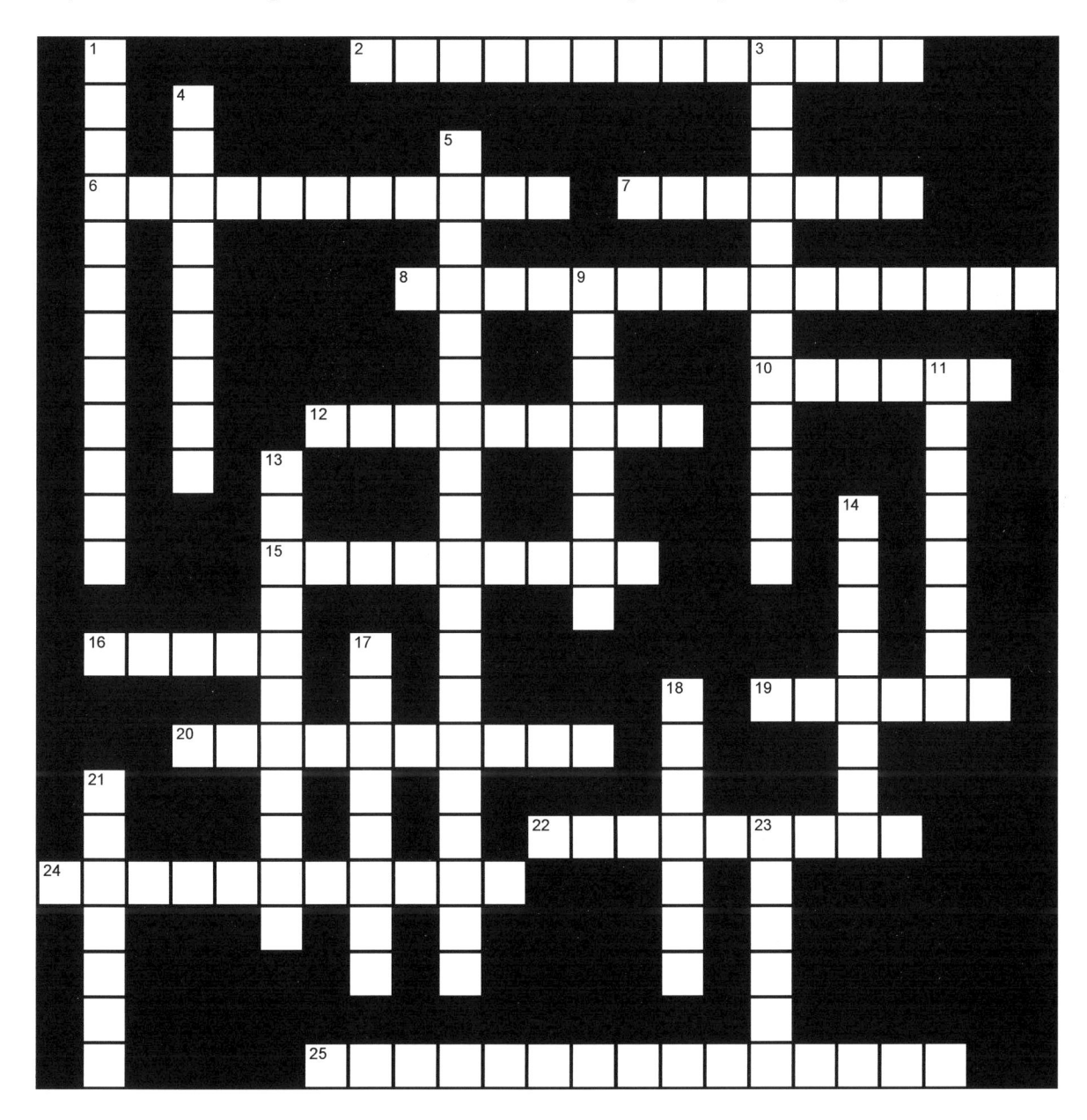

Across
2. During what phase of the menstrual cycle is oestrogen produced? (13)
6. The absence of menstruation (11)

Anatomy & Physiology Student Workbook

7. What glands secrete oestrogen and progesterone? (7)
8. Cushing's Syndrome is caused by the hypersecretion of what hormone? (15)
10. What does the hypersecretion of ADH cause? (6)
12. What hormone stimulates the breasts to produce milk following birth? (9)
15. What hormone is secreted by the pineal body? (9)
16. Where in the body can the pituitary gland be found? (5)
19. Mineralocorticoids and glucocorticoids are hormones secreted by what part of the adrenal glands? (6)
20. A stress hormone (10)
22. What gland is known as the master gland? (9)
24. What part of the nervous system is under the control of the adrenal medulla? (11)
25. What does the hyposecretion of mineralocorticoids cause? (15)

Down
1. What hormone is secreted by the parathyroid glands? (12)
3. What hormone controls the thyroid gland? (12)
4. What is caused by the hyposecretion of thyroxin? (9)
5. What hormone stimulates the testes to produce sperm? (19)
9. A hormone secreted by the posterior lobe of the pituitary gland (8)
11. The start of menstruation (8)
13. What hormone is responsible for controlling height and growth? (11)
14. What lobe of the pituitary gland secretes follicle stimulating hormone? (8)
17. What organ of the body contains the islets of langerhans that are responsible for producing insulin? (8)
18. Hypoglycaemia is caused by the hypersecretion of what hormone? (7)
21. What glands are positioned either side of the neck? (7)
23. Gland found in the thorax (6)

Exercise 5

In the table below, match the disease or disorder with the hyper/hyposecretion of various hormones. Please choose from the answers in the box at the end of this exercise.

1.	Hypersecretion of thyroid hormones	
2.	Hypersecretion of human growth hormone	
3.	Hypersecretion of glucocorticoids	
4.	Hyposecretion of insulin	
5.	Hyposecretion of parathormone	
6.	Hyposecretion of thyroid hormones	
7.	Hypersecretion of antidiuretic hormone	
8.	Hyposecretion of human growth hormone	
9.	Hypersecretion of mineralocorticoids	
10.	Hypersecretion of insulin	
11.	Hypersecretion of parathormone	
12.	Hyposecretion of mineralocorticoids	

Anatomy & Physiology Student Workbook

13.	Hypersecretion of oestrogen in men	
14.	Hypersecretion of testosterone in women	
15.	Hyposecretion of oestrogen in women	
16.	Hyposecretion of antidiuretic hormone	

Please choose your answers from the box below

Diabetes Mellitus	Tetany	Hypoglycaemia
Polycystic Ovarian Syndrome	Gynaecomastia	Gigantism
Kidney Failure	Dwarfism	Oedema
Cushing's Syndrome	Diabetes Insipidus	Softened Bones
Hirsutism	Cretinism	
Grave's Disease	Addison's Disease	

Exercise 6

In the table below, match the glands with where they are positioned in the body. Please choose your answers from the box at the end of this exercise.

1.	Either side of the neck		6.	Behind the thyroid	
2.	Centre of the brain		7.	Below the stomach	
3.	On top of each kidney		8.	Either side of the uterus	
4.	Within the scrotum		9.	In the thorax	
5.	Base of the brain				

Please choose the answers from the box below

Testes	Adrenal Glands	Ovaries
Thyroid Glands	Pancreas	Pineal Body
Pituitary Gland	Thymus	Parathyroid Glands

Exercise 7

Please answer the questions below and find the answers in the word search puzzle.

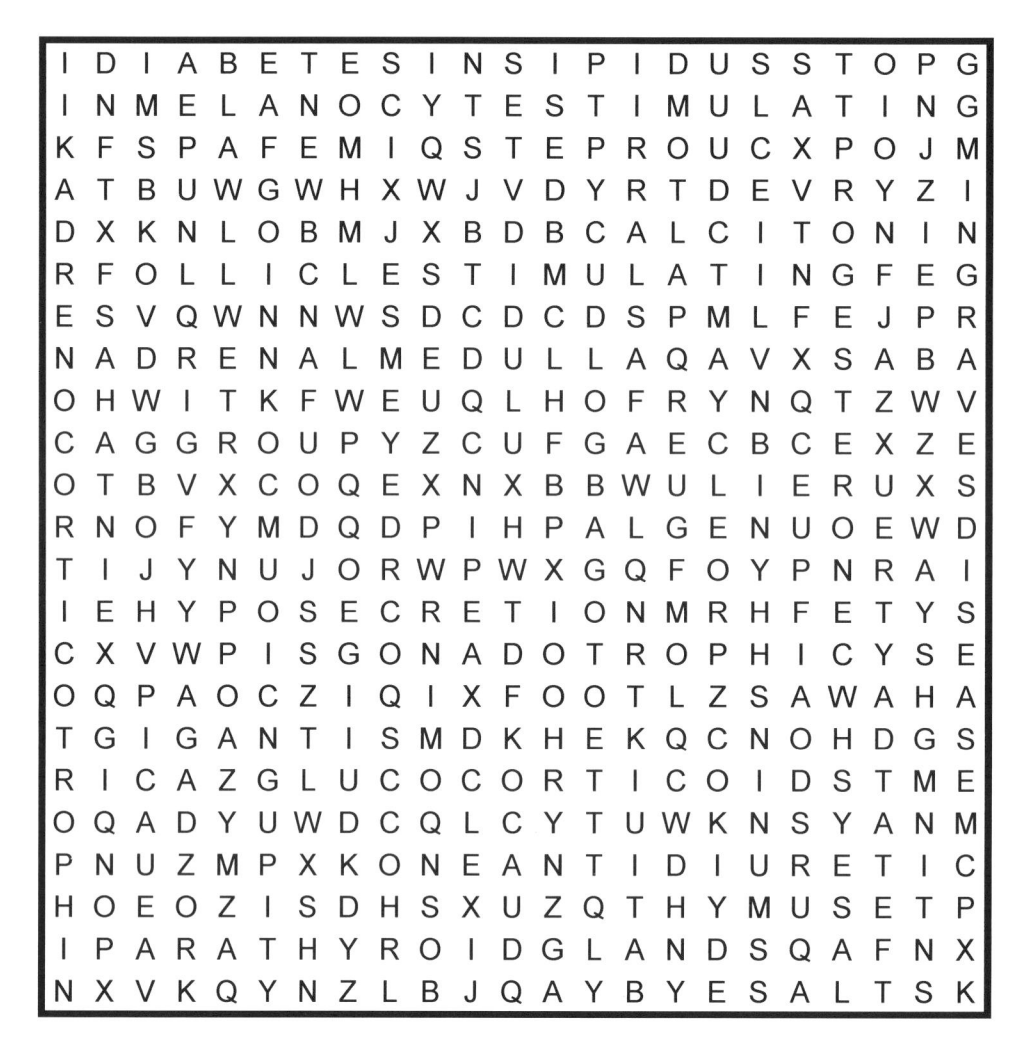

```
I D I A B E T E S I N S I P I D U S S T O P G
I N M E L A N O C Y T E S T I M U L A T I N G
K F S P A F E M I Q S T E P R O U C X P O J M
A T B U W G W H X W J V D Y R T D E V R Y Z I
D X K N L O B M J X B D B C A L C I T O N I N
R F O L L I C L E S T I M U L A T I N G F E G
E S V Q W N N W S D C D C D S P M L F E J P R
N A D R E N A L M E D U L L A Q A V X S A B A
O H W I T K F W E U Q L H O F R Y N Q T Z W V
C A G G R O U P Y Z C U F G A E C B C E X Z E
O T B V X C O Q E X N X B B W U L I E R U X S
R N O F Y M D Q D P I H P A L G E N U O E W D
T I J Y N U J O R W P W X G Q F O Y P N R A I
I E H Y P O S E C R E T I O N M R H F E T Y S
C X V W P I S G O N A D O T R O P H I C Y S E
O Q P A O C Z I Q I X F O O T L Z S A W A H A
T G I G A N T I S M D K H E K Q C N O H D G S
R I C A Z G L U C O C O R T I C O I D S T M E
O Q A D Y U W D C Q L C Y T U W K N S Y A N M
P N U Z M P X K O N E A N T I D I U R E T I C
H O E O Z I S D H S X U Z Q T H Y M U S E T P
I P A R A T H Y R O I D G L A N D S Q A F N X
N X V K Q Y N Z L B J Q A Y B Y E S A L T S K
```

1. What gland secretes adrenaline and noradrenaline? (14)
2. What endocrine gland is positioned below the stomach? (8)
3. What hormone of the anterior lobe of the pituitary gland stimulates the development of the graafian follicle in the ovary? (19)
4. TF and THF are hormones secreted by which gland? (6)
5. During what phase of the menstrual cycle does the hormone LH produce progesterone? (9)
6. What hormone is responsible for regulating female sexual development? (12)
7. What hormone controls the growth of the adrenal cortex? (20)
8. What does the hyposecretion of ADH cause? (17)
9. What is a chemical messenger? (7)
10. What does the hypersecretion of HGH cause? (9)
11. What hormone stimulates the production of melanin in the basal layer of the skin? (21)
12. What is caused by the hypersecretion of thyroxin? (13)
13. What hormone controls calcium levels in the blood? (10)

14. What hormone influences the digestion of carbohydrates, fats and proteins? (15)
15. What glands are positioned behind the thyroid glands? (17)
16. What hormone regulates water re absorption in the kidneys? (12)
17. The hormone responsible for controlling the development of the ovaries and testes (13)
18. What is regulated by mineralocorticoids? (5)
19. What hormone regulates blood sugar levels? (7)
20. Too little of any hormone secreted (13)

Exercise 8

Multiple choice questions, please choose one answer from the 4 choices provided in each box.

1. The effect of adrenaline on the body is; a) Decreases blood pressure b) Speeds up digestion c) Increase metabolic rate d) Dilates blood vessels Answer	2. Where is the thymus located? a) Thyroid glands b) Ovaries c) Thymus d) Top of kidneys Answer
3. The anterior and posterior lobes are part of which gland? a) Pituitary b) Thalamus c) Pancreas d) Adrenals Answer	4. The adrenal medulla is regulated by the; a) Sympathetic nervous system b) Central nervous system c) Somatic nervous system d) Parasympathetic nervous system Answer
5. Islets of Langerhans are found in; a) The liver b) The pancreas c) The adrenal glands d) The testes Answer	6. Hyposecretion of the thyroid gland hormones can lead to what disorder in an adult? a) Virilism b) Cretinism c) Addison's Disease d) Myxoedema Answer

7. What hormone increases the heart and breathing rates during times of stress? a) Insulin b) Adrenaline c) Glucocorticoids d) Oxytocin Answer _____	**8. What is the function of the endocrine system?** a) To produce hormones maintaining the body's functions b) To control changes to the body during pregnancy c) To control the body during stressful times d) All of the above Answer _____
9. What hormone is responsible for maintaining calcium levels in the body? a) Thyroxin b) Calcitonin c) Adrenaline d) Mineralocorticoids Answer _____	**10. Which one of the following hormones is not secreted by the anterior lobe of the pituitary gland?** a) Adrenocorticotrophin b) Thyrotrophin c) Antidiuretic hormone d) Melanocyte stimulating hormone Answer _____
11. Hypersecretion of mineralocorticoids causes; a) Addison's Disease b) Diabetes insipidus c) Kidney failure d) Cushing's syndrome Answer _____	**12. What is a hormone?** a) A ductless gland b) A blood vessel c) A chemical messenger d) A chemical catalyst Answer _____
13. What hormone controls the thyroid gland? a) Thyrotrophin b) Parathormone c) Thymic factor d) Glucocorticoids Answer _____	**14. What hormone is responsible for the growth of the female sexual characteristics?** a) Oestrogen b) Testosterone c) Insulin d) Luteinising hormone Answer _____

15. What hormone metabolises carbohydrates, proteins and fats? a) Mineralocorticoids b) Thyrotrophin c) Adrenaline d) Glucocorticoids Answer	**16. Hyposecretion of insulin causes;** a) Diabetes mellitus b) Hypoglycaemia c) Diabetes insipidus d) Grave's disease Answer
17. What hormone is secreted by the pineal body? a) Oxytocin b) Melatonin c) Insulin d) Gonadotrophins Answer	**18. During what phase of the menstrual cycle does ovulation occur?** a) Menarche b) Menstrual c) Proliferative d) Secretory Answer
19. A condition called tetany occurs when there is; a) A deficiency of blood sugar in the blood b) A deficiency of calcium in the blood c) A deficiency of vitamin A in the blood d) A deficiency of salts in the blood Answer	**20. Which one of the following is not a function of the thyroid gland?** a) Regulates basic metabolic rate b) Maintains healthy skin and hair c) Increases water reabsorption in the kidneys d) Controls the rate at which the body's cells work Answer
21. Hypersecretion of testosterone in females can lead to; a) SAD b) Hirsutism c) Polycystic Ovarian Syndrome d) Gynaecomastia Answer	**22. What is the definition of amenorrhoea?** a) Painful menstruation b) The start of the menstrual cycle c) The onset of menopause d) The absence of menstruation Answer

23. What hormone is secreted when the body finds itself in an emergency situation?
a) Adrenaline
b) Insulin
c) Glycogen
d) Glucocorticoids

Answer

24. Which one of the following is not a phase of the menstrual cycle?
a) Menarche
b) Secretory
c) Menstrual
d) Proliferative

Answer

25. What are the effects of grave's disease?
a) Decreased heart and breathing rates
b) Increase heart rate and disturbed sleeping patterns
c) Low blood pressure and oedema
d) Depression and weight gain

Answer

26. What endocrine gland is located below the stomach?
a) Ovaries
b) Pineal body
c) Adrenal medulla
d) Pancreas

Answer

27. What is the function of HGH?
a) To control the thyroid gland
b) To control salt levels in the blood
c) To regulate height and growth
d) To regulate water reabsorption

Answer

28. What hormone is secreted by the pancreas?
a) Melatonin
b) Adrenaline
c) Parathormone
d) Insulin

Answer

29. What hormone stimulates the production of sperm in men?
a) Follicle stimulating hormone
b) Luteinising hormone
c) Prolactin
d) Oxytocin

Answer

30. What is the function of melanocyte stimulating hormone?
a) To stimulate the basal layer of the skin to produce melanin
b) To stimulate the clear layer of skin to produce melanin
c) To stimulate the surface layer of the skin to produce melanin
d) To stimulate the dermis to produce melanin

Answer

31. Antidiuretic hormone is secreted by the; a) Pancreas b) Anterior lobe of the pituitary gland c) Posterior lobe of the pituitary gland d) Adrenal cortex Answer	**32. Hypoglycaemia is a term used to describe;** a) High blood pressure b) Low blood pressure c) High blood sugar d) Low blood sugar Answer
33. Which one of the following hormones is secreted by the anterior lobe of the pituitary gland? a) TF b) ADH c) Vasopressin d) HGH Answer	**34. What endocrine gland is located in the centre of the brain?** a) Parathyroid gland b) Pineal body c) Adrenal cortex d) Pituitary gland Answer
35. What is the function of parathyroid glands? a) To regulate salt levels in the body b) To regulate calcium levels in the blood c) To metabolise carbohydrates and proteins d) To regulate blood sugar levels Answer	**36. Muscular weakness and changes in skin pigmentation are effects of what endocrine disorder?** a) Myxoedema b) Addison's syndrome c) Gigantism d) Amenorrhoea Answer
37. What type of diabetes occurs as a result of the pancreas being unable to produce insulin? a) Cushings b) Insipidus c) Mellitus d) Acromegaly Answer	**38. What is the function of oxytocin?** a) To stimulate the contraction of the uterus during labour b) To prepare the corpus luteum for pregnancy c) To stimulate the ovaries to produce oestrogen d) To control sexual development in females Answer

| 39. Hypersecretion of glucocorticoids causes;
 a) Diabetes mellitus <br> b) Cushing's syndrome <br> c) Addison's disease <br> d) Amenorrhoea

 Answer _____ | 40. Where is the pituitary gland located?
 a) Below the stomach <br> b) Front of the neck <br> c) Base of the brain <br> d) Centre of the brain

 Answer _____ |

The Endocrine System
Answers

Exercise 1 (true/false):
1. True	11. False	21. True	31. True
2. False	12. True	22. True	32. True
3. False	13. False	23. False	33. False
4. False	14. True	24. False	34. False
5. True	15. True	25. True	35. True
6. False	16. False	26. True	36. True
7. True	17. True	27. True	37. False
8. False	18. True	28. False	38. False
9. True	19. False	29. False	39. True
10. False	20. False	30. True	40. False

Exercise 2 (match the endocrine glands with the hormones they secrete):
1. Anterior Lobe of the Pituitary Gland
2. Pineal Body
3. Adrenal Cortex
4. Testes
5. Thyroid Glands
6. Adrenal Medulla
7. Anterior Lobe of the Pituitary Gland
8. Thyroid Glands
9. Ovaries
10. Pancreas
11. Anterior Lobe of the Pituitary Gland
12. Parathyroid Glands
13. Anterior Lobe of the Pituitary Gland
14. Adrenal Medulla
15. Thyroid Glands
16. Posterior Lobe of the Pituitary Gland
17. Adrenal Cortex
18. Ovaries
19. Thymus
20. Anterior Lobe of the Pituitary Gland
21. Posterior Lobe of the Pituitary Gland
22. Anterior Lobe of the Pituitary Gland

Exercise 3 (fill in the missing words):
1. Ductless
2. Metabolic
3. Bloodstream
4. Anterior
5. Medulla
6. Melatonin
7. Chemical
8. Water
9. Thyroid
10. Hyposecretion
11. Proliferative
12. Testosterone
13. Kidney
14. Posterior
15. Myxoedema

Exercise 4 (crossword):

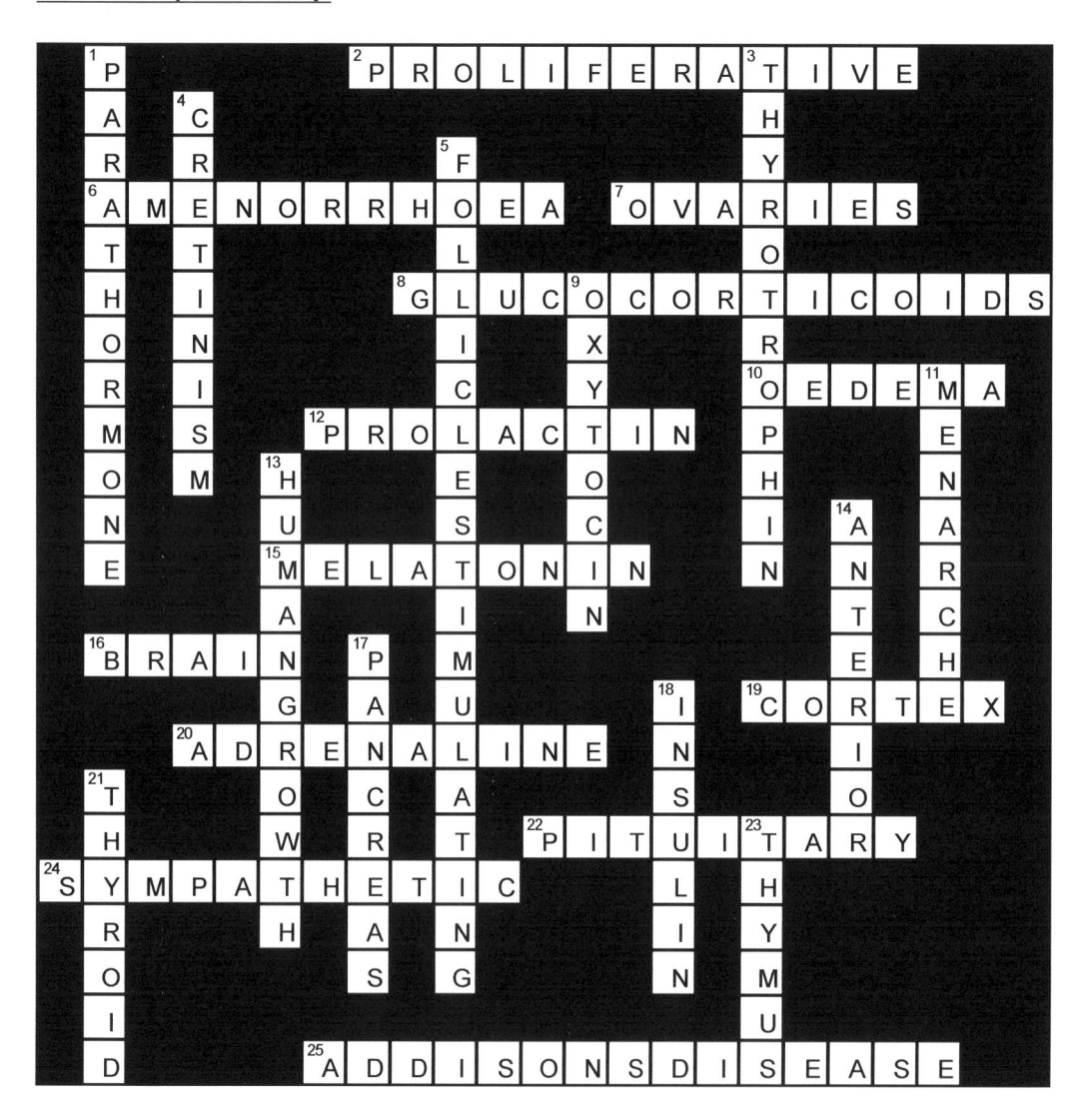

Exercise 5 (match the disease/disorders with the hyper/hyposecretion of hormones):

1. Grave's Disease
2. Gigantism
3. Cushing's Syndrome
4. Diabetes Mellitus
5. Tetany
6. Cretinism
7. Oedema
8. Dwarfism
9. Kidney Failure
10. Hypoglycaemia
11. Softened Bones
12. Addison's Disease
13. Gynaecomastia
14. Hirsutism
15. Polycystic Ovarian Syndrome
16. Diabetes Insipidus

Exercise 6 (match the glands with their positions in the body):

1. Thyroid Glands
2. Pineal Body
3. Adrenal Glands
4. Testes
5. Pituitary
6. Parathyroid Glands
7. Pancreas
8. Ovaries
9. Thymus

Exercise 7 (word search):

1. Adrenal Medulla
2. Pancreas
3. Follicle Stimulating
4. Thymus
5. Secretory
6. Progesterone
7. Adrenocorticotrophin
8. Diabetes Insipidus
9. Hormone
10. Gigantism
11. Melanocyte Stimulating
12. Grave's Disease
13. Calcitonin
14. Glucocorticoids
15. Parathyroid Glands
16. Antidiuretic
17. Gonadotrophic
18. Salts
19. Insulin
20. Hyposecretion

Exercise 8 (multiple choice questions):

1	C	9	B	17	B	25	B	33	D
2	C	10	C	18	C	26	D	34	B
3	A	11	C	19	B	27	C	35	B
4	A	12	C	20	C	28	D	36	B
5	B	13	A	21	B	29	A	37	C
6	D	14	A	22	D	30	A	38	A
7	B	15	D	23	A	31	C	39	B
8	D	16	A	24	A	32	D	40	C

Chapter 8 | The Nervous System

Revision Puzzles & Questions

Exercise 1

The following grid lists statements on the left that are either true or false. Please choose your answer on the right. All answers are provided at the end of the chapter.

1.	The peripheral nervous system consists of the brain and the spinal cord	True ☐ False ☐
2.	Neurones conduct nerve impulses	True ☐ False ☐
3.	The myelin sheath is a fatty substance surrounding the synapse	True ☐ False ☐
4.	The dura mater is the outer protective layer of the meninges	True ☐ False ☐
5.	Motor nerves are also known as efferent nerves	True ☐ False ☐
6.	The cardiac centre is found in the medulla oblongata	True ☐ False ☐
7.	There are 12 pairs of cervical nerves	True ☐ False ☐

Anatomy & Physiology Student Workbook

8.	Neurons produce acetylcholine	True ☐ False ☐
9.	The sympathetic nervous system slows down the heart rate	True ☐ False ☐
10.	The sacral plexus supply the muscles and skin of the shoulder and upper chest	True ☐ False ☐
11.	The hypothalamus regulates hunger and thirst	True ☐ False ☐
12.	The midbrain is part of the brain stem	True ☐ False ☐
13.	The cerebellum is responsible for controlling decision making	True ☐ False ☐
14.	Nodes of ranvier are gaps in the myelin sheath along the length of the axon	True ☐ False ☐
15.	The axon is responsible for supporting and protecting the neurones	True ☐ False ☐
16.	Cerebrospinal fluid forms a cushion between the spinal and cranial nerves	True ☐ False ☐
17.	A reflex action requires only an afferent neurone for a movement to take place	True ☐ False ☐

18.	The cerebrum is the largest part of the brain	True ☐ False ☐
19.	The outer layer of the cerebrum is called the cerebral cortex	True ☐ False ☐
20.	There are 12 pairs of spinal nerves	True ☐ False ☐
21.	The parasympathetic nervous system prepares the body for stressful or emergency situations	True ☐ False ☐
22.	The cervical plexus supplies the muscles of the head and neck	True ☐ False ☐
23.	The cerebrum regulates memory	True ☐ False ☐
24.	The 4 lobes of the cerebellum include frontal, temporal, parietal and occipital	True ☐ False ☐
25.	The medulla oblongata is known as the vital centre of the brain	True ☐ False ☐
26.	The spinal cord transmits messages to and from the brain	True ☐ False ☐
27.	Grey matter is found on the outside of the spinal cord and inside the brain	True ☐ False ☐

28.	The cell body is found in the centre of the neuroglia	True ☐ False ☐
29.	Neuroglia help to provide support and protection for the neurones	True ☐ False ☐
30.	Mixed neurones contain sensory and motor nerves	True ☐ False ☐
31.	Dendrites transmit nerve impulses towards the cell body	True ☐ False ☐
32.	The somatic nervous system is controlled by the hypothalamus	True ☐ False ☐
33.	The peripheral nervous system is divided into the somatic and autonomic nervous systems	True ☐ False ☐
34.	The brain stem consists of the pons varolii, midbrain and the medulla oblongata	True ☐ False ☐
35.	The pons varolii maintains the balance and equilibrium of the body	True ☐ False ☐
36.	Neurilemma is a membrane which surrounds the axon and is found in the brain and spinal cord	True ☐ False ☐
37.	Multiple sclerosis occurs when the protective myelin sheath is destroyed	True ☐ False ☐

38.	Facial paralysis is the result of bell's palsy	True ☐ False ☐
39.	The hypothalamus controls the actions of the heart and lungs	True ☐ False ☐
40.	The olfactory nerve is a sensory nerve of smell	True ☐ False ☐

Exercise 2

In the table below, match the spinal plexus nerves with the body parts that they supply. Please note, some spinal nerves may be repeated.

1.	Diaphragm		6.	Pelvic Area	
2.	Lower Leg		7.	Upper Chest	
3.	Arm		8.	Neck	
4.	Groin		9.	Hand	
5.	Coccyx		10.	Thighs	

Please choose the answers from the box below

Sacral	Cervical
Coccygeal	Brachial
Brachial	Lumbar
Lumbar	Sacral
Brachial	Cervical

Exercise 3

Complete the following crossword on The Nervous System by answering the clues below.

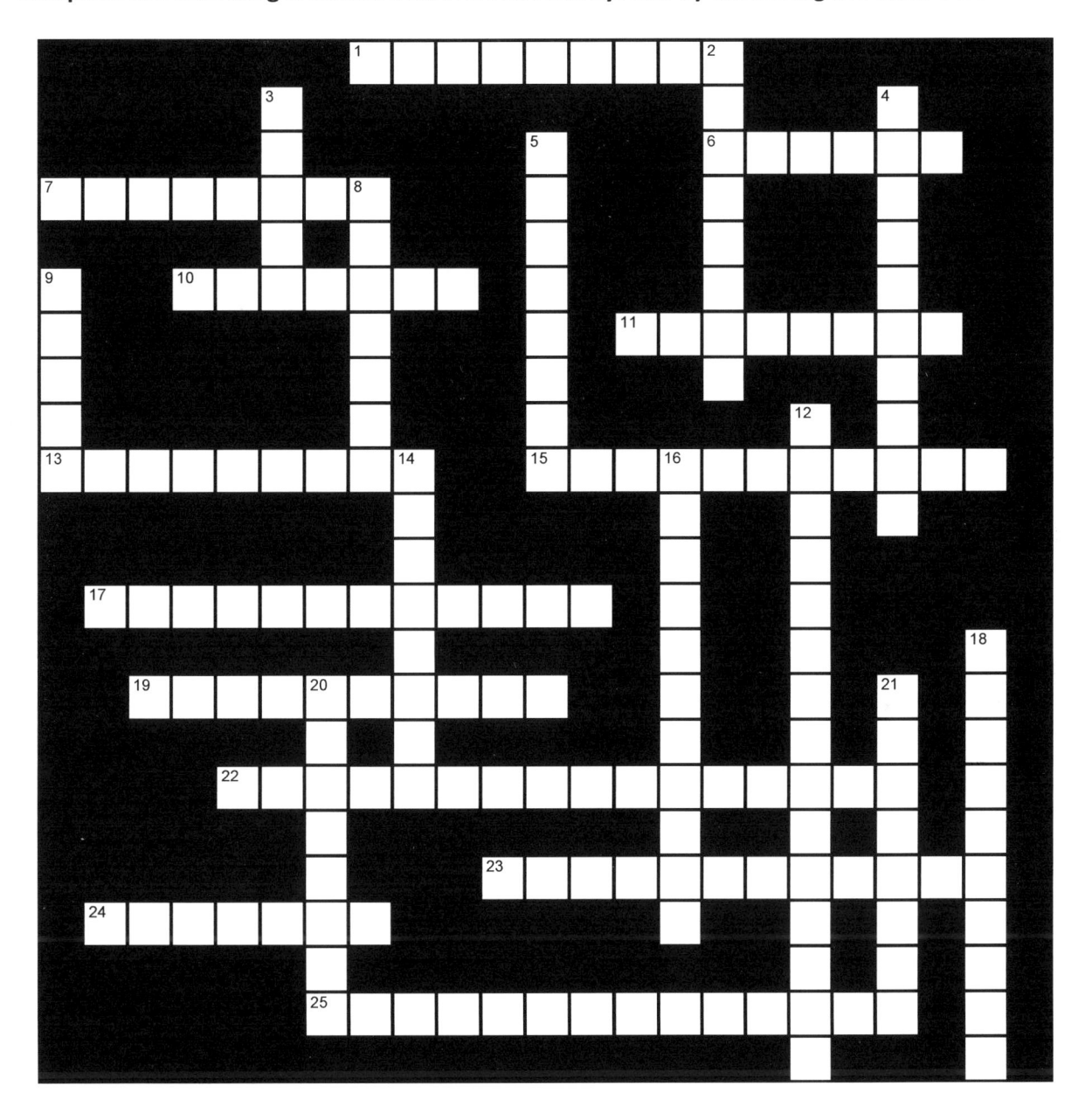

Across
1. What part of the nervous system is divided into the sympathetic and parasympathetic nervous systems (9)
6. What is an automatic instinctive reaction to a sensory stimulus? (6)
7. Inflammation of a nerve (8)
10. What nerve supplies the diaphragm allowing it to move? (7)
11. What is another name for nerve cells? (8)
13. What are nerve fibres that transmit nerve impulses towards the cell body? (9)

15. What does the hypothalamus help to regulate within the body? (11)
17. What part of the brain regulates the pituitary gland? (12)
19. What substance in the brain consists of neuronal cell bodies and dendrites (10)
22. What part of the brain is known as the vital centre (16)
23. What protective sheath covers the axon? (12)
24. The somatic nervous system contains 12 pairs of nerves, what are they called? (7)
25. What part of the neurone increases the speed at which nerve impulses pass along the fibre? (14)

Down
2. What part of the brain controls memory? (8)
3. Another name for efferent nerves (5)
4. What part of the brain is known as the small brain? (10)
5. What nerves transmit impulses towards the brain? (8)
8. What is the point where one neurone meets another? (7)
9. What type of nerves, transmit motor and sensory nerve fibres? (5)
12. What part of the autonomic nervous system slows down heart & breathing rates? (15)
14. What type of muscular activity is regulated by the cerebellum? (8)
16. What part of the brain stem bridges the hemispheres of the cerebellum? (11)
18. What nervous system consists of the cranial and spinal nerves? (10)
20. What part of the brain acts as a relay station for visual and auditory information? (8)
21. What part of the meninges supply blood to the brain and spinal cord? (8)

Exercise 4

In the table, match what parts of the brain are responsible for controlling the functions listed below. The 5 parts of the brain that you must choose from are: 1. Cerebrum 2. Cerebellum 3. Medulla Oblongata 4. Hypothalamus 5. Midbrain.

1.	Voluntary Movement		14.	Co-ordination of eye movements	
2.	Sneezing		15.	Heart's Actions	
3.	Memory		16.	Hearing	
4.	Muscle Tone		17.	Hunger	
5.	Dilation of blood vessels		18.	Skeletal Muscular Activity	
6.	Balance		19.	Thirst	
7.	Reasoning		20.	Sex Drive	
8.	Swallowing		21.	Body Temperature	
9.	Touch		22.	Posture	
10.	Vomiting		23.	Vision	
11.	Smell		24.	Sleep Patterns	

12.	Rate of Breathing		25.	Hormones	
13.	Taste				

Exercise 5

Please answer the questions below and find the answers in the word search puzzle.

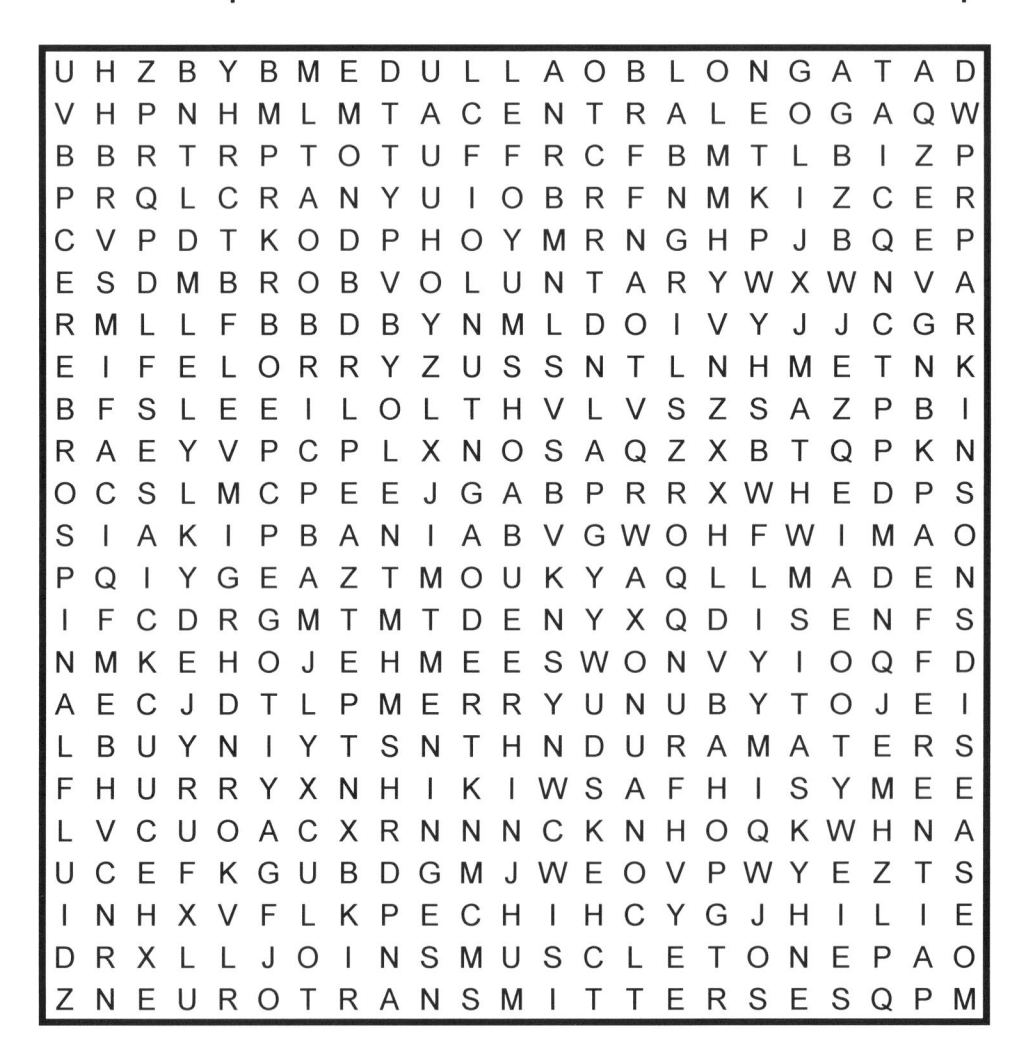

```
U H Z B Y B M E D U L L A O B L O N G A T A D
V H P N H M L M T A C E N T R A L E O G A Q W
B B R T R P T O T U F F R C F B M T L B I Z P
P R Q L C R A N Y U I O B R F N M K I Z C E R
C V P D T K O D P H O Y M R N G H P J B Q E P
E S D M B R O B V O L U N T A R Y W X W N V A
R M L L F B B D B Y N M L D O I V Y J J C G R
E I F E L O R R Y Z U S S N T L N H M E T N K
B F S L E E I L O L T H V L V S Z S A Z P B I
R A E Y V P C P L X N O S A Q Z X B T Q P K N
O C S L M C P E E J G A B P R R X W H E D P S
S I A K I P B A N I A B V G W O H F W I M A O
P Q I Y G E A Z T M O U K Y A Q L L M A D E N
I F C D R G M T M T D E N Y X Q D I S E N F S
N M K E H O J E H M E E S W O N V Y I O Q F D
A E C J D T L P M E R R Y U N U B Y T O J E I
L B U Y N I Y T S N T H N D U R A M A T E R S
F H U R R Y X N H I K I W S A F H I S Y M E E
L V C U O A C X R N N N C K N H O Q K W H N A
U C E F K G U B D G M J W E O V P W Y E Z T S
I N H X V F L K P E C H I H C Y G J H I L I E
D R X L L J O I N S M U S C L E T O N E P A O
Z N E U R O T R A N S M I T T E R S E S Q P M
```

1. What part of the brain consists of the midbrain, pons varolii and medulla oblongata? (9)
2. What connects the brain with the spinal cord? (16)
3. What membrane, made up of connective tissue, protects the central nervous system? (8)
4. What part of the autonomic nervous system prepares the body to deal with emergency situations? (11)

5. What fine, thin membrane surrounds the myelin sheath? (10)
6. What are the chemicals called that are released by the nerve endings? (17)
7. What bodily function is controlled by the hypothalamus (13)
8. What part of the brain is responsible for the balance of the body (10)
9. What part of the nervous system consists of the brain and spinal cord? (7)
10. What disease of the nervous system is caused by damage to basal ganglia of the brain? (17)
11. What is the outer layer of the meninges called? (9)
12. What fluid protects the brain and spinal cord by acting as a shock absorber? (18)
13. What is the centre of a neurone called? (8)
14. The long single nerve fibre that transmits nerve impulses away from the cell body (4)
15. What type of nerves carry impulses from the brain or spinal cord? (8)
16. What type of movement is the cerebrum responsible for controlling? (9)
17. What is the cerebellum responsible for controlling? (10)
18. What form of connective tissue supports and protects the neurones? (9)
19. A lobe of the cerebrum (7)
20. Part of the brain stem (11)

Exercise 6

Fill in the missing words.

1. There are _____ pairs of cranial nerves in the peripheral nervous system (2)

2. The sympathetic nervous system _____ the heart rate (9)

3. Sensory neurones are also known as _____ neurones (8)

4. The peripheral nervous system is divided into the somatic and _____ nervous systems (9)

5. The _____ _____ speeds up movement of nerve impulses along the axon's length (6,6)

6. The cerebrum is the _____ part of the brain (7)

7. The autonomic nervous system is regulated by the _____ (12)

8. The brachial plexuses supply the _____ chest (5)

9. _____ is caused by the inflammation of the meninges (10)

10. The _____ mater is positioned underneath the dura mater (9)

11. The medulla oblongata contains control centres for the _____ and lungs (5)

12. Dendrites receive and transmit messages _____ the cell body (7)

13. Cerebrospinal fluid carries _____ away from the nerve tissue (5)

14. The _____ _____ allows communication to take place between the hemispheres of the cerebrum (6,8)

15. The olfactory nerve is the sensory nerve of _____ (5)

16. The _____ nervous system prepares the body for highly stressful situations (11)

17. _____ _____ occurs when the myelin sheath around nerve fibres is destroyed (8,9)

18. The _____ carries impulses away from the cell body (4)

19. Neurones and _____ are 2 types of nervous tissue (9)

20. The _____ _____ is a layer of the cerebrum where most functions are carried out (8,6)

Exercise 7

Multiple choice questions, please choose one answer from the 4 choices provided in each box.

1. Which one of the following is not a type of neurone? a) Afferent b) Motor c) Mixed d) Axon Answer	2. How many pairs of cranial nerves does the somatic nervous system contain? a) 12 b) 17 c) 31 d) 28 Answer
3. Which one of the following is not a lobe of the cerebrum? a) Temoral b) Parietal c) Occipital d) Lacrimal Answer	4. Which one of the following is not a function of the sympathetic nervous system? a) Increases heart rate b) Decreases breathing rate c) Increases the volume of circulating blood d) Vasodilation of skeletal blood vessels Answer
5. Where is the mitochondria found in a nerve cell? a) Cell body b) Axon c) Nucleus d) Nodes of ranvier Answer	6. What part of the brain regulates the pituitary gland? a) Hypothalamus b) Pons varolii c) Cerebellum d) Midbrain Answer
7. What plexus supplies the pelvic area? a) Lumbar b) Brachial c) Sacral d) Thoracic Answer	8. What part of the brain is found at the back of the cranium? a) Cerebellum b) Cerebrum c) Hypothalamus d) Pons varolii Answer

9. Which one of the following is the inner layer of the meninges
a) Dura
b) Pia
c) Associated
d) Arachnoid

Answer
_____

10. What is the function of the spinal cord?
a) It transmits impulses to and from the brain
b) It transmits impulses away from the brain
c) It transmits impulses to all parts of the body
d) It transmits impulses to the nerves of the body

Answer
_____

11. What disease of the nervous system affects motor system control?
a) Cerebral palsy
b) Sciatica
c) Bell's palsy
d) Meningitis

Answer
_____

12. What part of the nerve fibre contains important organelles?
a) Neurilemma
b) Cell body
c) Nodes of ranvier
d) Axon

Answer
_____

13. What substance is found on the inside of the brain?
a) White matter
b) Unmyelinated sheath
c) Endothelial cells
d) Grey matter

Answer
_____

14. Efferent nerves are another term for;
a) Sensory
b) Afferent
c) Motor
d) Mixed

Answer
_____

15. What is the function of cerebrospinal fluid?
a) To transmit messages to the spinal cord
b) To supply the brain with oxygen
c) To supply nerve impulses to the diaphragm instructing it to contract
d) It carries waste substances away from the nerve tissue

Answer
_____

16. What part of the neurone transmits impulses away from the cell body?
a) Myelin sheath
b) Axon
c) Dendrites
d) Synapse

Answer
_____

17. What is the outer layer of the cerebrum called? a) Dura mater b) Corpus callosum c) Cerebral cortex d) Midbrain Answer	18. What part of the brain regulates the autonomic nervous system? a) Hypothalamus b) Midbrain c) Medulla oblongata d) Cerebellum Answer
19. What part of the brain controls mental activity? a) Hypothalamus b) Medulla oblongata c) Cerebellum d) Cerebrum Answer	20. The point at which nerve impulses pass from one neurone to the next; a) Dendrites b) Nodes of ranvier c) Axon d) Synapse Answer
21. Which one of the following is not part of the brain stem? a) Midbrain b) Medulla oblongata c) Hypothalamus d) Pons varolii Answer	22. What part of the brain controls vomiting and coughing? a) Hypothalamus b) Medulla oblongata c) Cerebellum d) Cerebrum Answer
23. What part of the nervous system do the meninges not protect? a) Sympathetic b) Medulla oblongata c) Pons varolii d) Cerebellum Answer	24. Which one of the following is not a cranial nerve of the eye? a) Oculomotor b) Trochlear c) Optic d) Olfactory Answer

Anatomy & Physiology Student Workbook

25. Which one of the following is a continuation of the spinal cord? a) Midbrain b) Pons varolii c) Medulla oblongata d) Hypothalamus Answer	**26. What is the function of the midbrain?** a) It controls the action of the heart b) It controls voluntary movements c) It controls the muscle tone of the body d) It controls visual and auditory systems Answer
27. What type of neurones stimulate muscles to produce movement? a) Sensory b) Axon c) Afferent d) Motor Answer	**28. How many pairs of spinal nerves are there?** a) 12 b) 7 c) 5 d) 8 Answer
29. What is the function of dendrites? a) To protect the axon b) Transmit nerve impulses away from the cell body c) Transmit impulses from the spinal cord to the brain d) Transmit nerve impulses towards the cell body Answer	**30. Glial cells are another term for;** a) Nodes of ranvier b) Neurones c) Neuroglia d) Neurilemma Answer
31. What is the corpus callosum? a) Nerve fibres bridging the hemispheres of the cerebellum b) Nerve fibres bridging the hemispheres of the cerebrum c) Nerve fibres bridging the hemispheres of the medulla oblongata d) Nerve fibres bridging the hemispheres of the hypothalamus Answer	**32. Which one of the following is not controlled by the hypothalamus?** a) Appetite b) Regulation of body temperature c) Voluntary movements d) Sleep patterns Answer

33. Which one of the following is part of the brain stem?	34. What part of the nerve cell accelerates the rate at which messages are transmitted?
a) Pons varolii b) Hypothalamus c) Cerebral cortex d) Cerebellum Answer	a) Dendrites b) Axon c) Myelin sheath d) Synapse Answer
35. What is the function of the medulla oblongata?	36. What is the function of neurones?
a) To control swallowing b) To control memory c) To control voluntary movement d) To control appetite Answer	a) To conduct electrical and chemical impulses throughout the nervous system b) To conduct sensory stimuli across the axon terminal c) To transmit impulses to and from the peripheral nervous system d) To carry messages across the corpus callosum Answer
37. What nervous system supplies impulses to smooth muscle?	38. Which one of the following is not controlled by the cerebellum?
a) Somatic b) Autonomic c) Central d) Nervous Answer	a) Balance b) Muscle tone c) Co-ordination of skeletal muscles d) Dilation of blood vessels Answer
39. What layer of the meninges is filled with cerebrospinal fluid?	40. The point at which impulses pass from one neurone to the next;
a) Pia b) Arachnoid c) Dura d) Fibrous Answer	a) Axon terminals b) Synapse c) Neurilemma d) Dendrites Answer

The Nervous System
Answers

Exercise 1 (true/false):

1. False	11. True	21. False	31. True
2. True	12. True	22. True	32. False
3. False	13. False	23. True	33. True
4. True	14. True	24. False	34. True
5. True	15. False	25. True	35. False
6. True	16. False	26. True	36. False
7. False	17. False	27. False	37. True
8. True	18. True	28. False	38. True
9. False	19. True	29. True	39. False
10. False	20. False	30. True	40. True

Exercise 2 (match the spinal plexus nerves with the parts of the body they supply):

1. Cervical
2. Sacral
3. Brachial
4. Lumbar
5. Coccygeal
6. Sacral
7. Brachial
8. Cervical
9. Brachial
10. Lumbar

Exercise 3 (crossword):

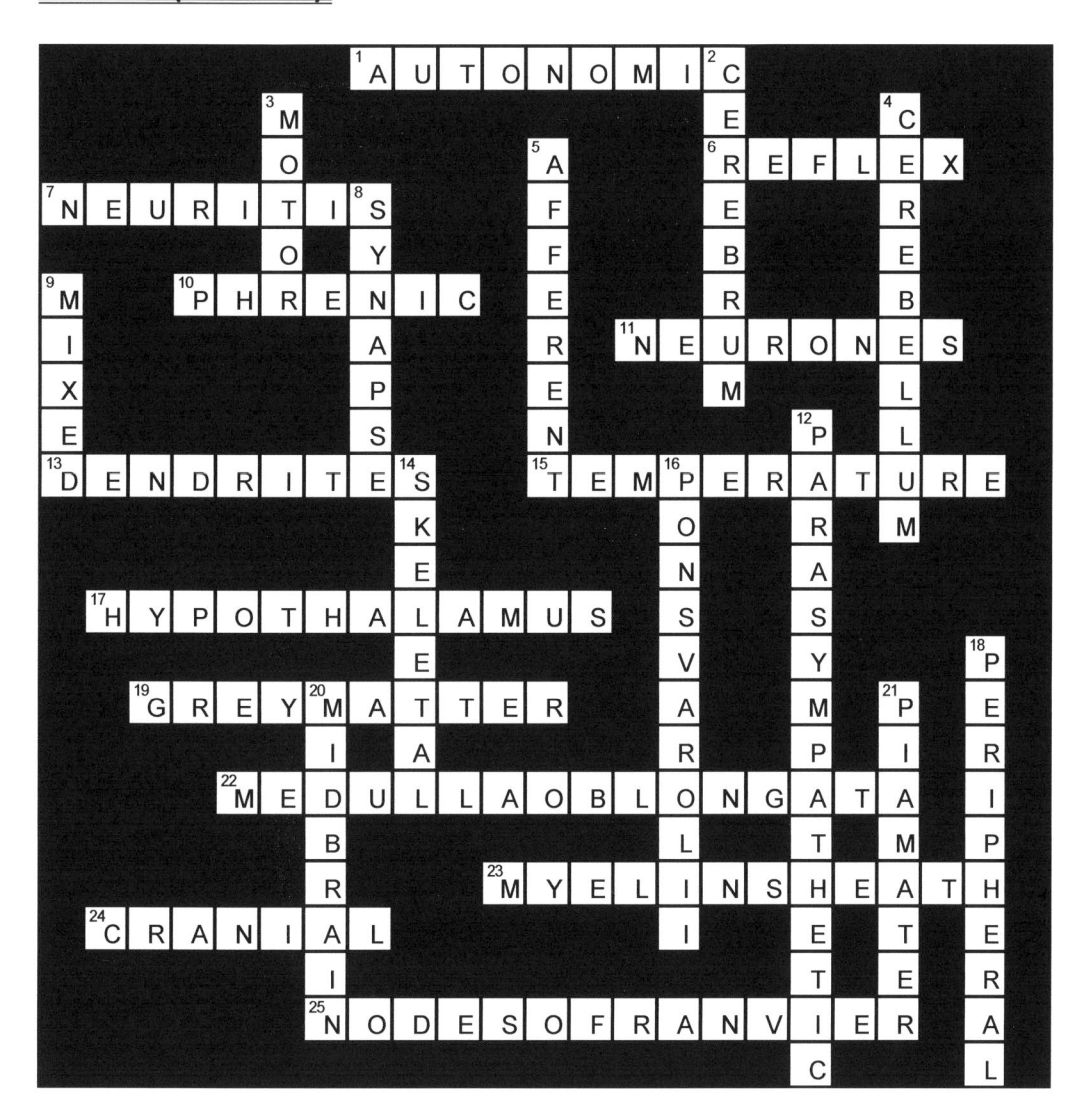

Exercise 4 (match the parts of the brain with their corresponding functions):

1. Cerebrum
2. Medulla Oblongata
3. Cerebrum
4. Cerebellum
5. Medulla Oblongata
6. Cerebellum
7. Cerebrum
8. Medulla Oblongata
9. Cerebrum
10. Medulla Oblongata
11. Cerebrum
12. Medulla Oblongata
13. Cerebrum
14. Midbrain
15. Medulla Oblongata
16. Cerebrum
17. Hypothalamus
18. Cerebellum
19. Hypothalamus
20. Hypothalamus
21. Hypothalamus
22. Cerebellum
23. Cerebrum
24. Hypothalamus
25. Hypothalamus

Exercise 5 (word search):

1. Brain Stem
2. Medulla Oblongata
3. Meninges
4. Sympathetic
5. Neurilemma
6. Neurotransmitters
7. Sleep Patterns
8. Cerebellum
9. Central
10. Parkinson's Disease
11. Dura Mater
12. Cerebrospinal Fluid
13. Cell Body
14. Axon
15. Efferent
16. Voluntary
17. Muscle Tone
18. Neuroglia
19. Frontal
20. Pons Varolii

Exercise 6 (fill in the missing words):

1. 12
2. Increases
3. Afferent
4. Autonomic
5. Myelin sheath
6. Largest
7. Hypothalamus
8. Upper
9. Meningitis
10. Arachnoid
11. Heart
12. Towards
13. Waste
14. Corpus Callosum
15. Smell
16. Sympathetic
17. Multiple Sclerosis
18. Axon
19. Neuroglia
20. Cerebral Cortex

Exercise 7 (multiple choice questions):

1	D	9	B	17	C	25	C	33	A
2	A	10	A	18	A	26	D	34	C
3	D	11	A	19	D	27	D	35	A
4	B	12	B	20	D	28	C	36	A
5	A	13	A	21	C	29	D	37	B
6	A	14	C	22	B	30	C	38	D
7	C	15	D	23	A	31	B	39	B
8	A	16	B	24	D	32	C	40	B

Chapter 9 | The Reproductive System

Revision Puzzles & Questions

Exercise 1

The following grid lists statements on the left that are either true or false. Please choose your answer on the right. All answers are provided at the end of the chapter.

1.	The breast is made up of lymphoid tissue	True ☐ False ☐
2.	The Cowper's glands open into the urethra at the base of the penis	True ☐ False ☐
3.	Painful menstruation is known as amenorrhoea	True ☐ False ☐
4.	The labia majora are folds of skin within the labia minora that protect the clitoris	True ☐ False ☐
5.	The uterus is another name for the womb	True ☐ False ☐
6.	Immature sperm cells are stored within the epididymis	True ☐ False ☐
7.	The cervix is the first part of the birth canal	True ☐ False ☐

Anatomy & Physiology Student Workbook

8.	The prostate gland leads from the epididymis to the urethra	True ☐ False ☐
9.	The perimetrium is the outer layer of the uterus	True ☐ False ☐
10.	The fertilised ovum is called the embryo	True ☐ False ☐
11.	The tip of the penis is known as the peritoneum	True ☐ False ☐
12.	The testes are the male gonads	True ☐ False ☐
13.	The fallopian tubes transport the ovum from the ovary to the vagina	True ☐ False ☐
14.	The head of the sperm carries the chromosomes	True ☐ False ☐
15.	The zygote contains 46 chromosomes	True ☐ False ☐
16.	The vas deferens leads from the epididymis to the urethra	True ☐ False ☐
17.	A fibroid is an abnormal growth of areolar connective tissue and muscular tissue	True ☐ False ☐

18.	The top end of the uterus opens into the vagina	True ☐ False ☐
19.	Fertilisation of the ovum takes place within the fallopian tubes	True ☐ False ☐
20.	Mitotic cell division of the zygote results in a mass of cells called the morula	True ☐ False ☐
21.	The endometrium is the outer membrane lining of the ovaries	True ☐ False ☐
22.	The cardiovascular system begins to develop in the second month of pregnancy	True ☐ False ☐
23.	The ovaries are the female gonads	True ☐ False ☐
24.	The function of the prostate gland is to produce sperm	True ☐ False ☐
25.	The vas deferens carries sperm from the epididymis to the ureter	True ☐ False ☐
26.	During a hysterectomy the uterus is removed	True ☐ False ☐
27.	The embryo becomes the foetus from 8 weeks	True ☐ False ☐

28.	Glans is another name for foreskin	True ☐ False ☐
29.	Mature follicles on the surface of the ovaries are known as graafian follicles	True ☐ False ☐
30.	A blastocyst implants in the lining of the uterus on day 24	True ☐ False ☐
31.	Absence of menstruation is known as amenorrhoea	True ☐ False ☐
32.	Parturition is another term used to describe giving birth	True ☐ False ☐
33.	The testes are contained within the penis	True ☐ False ☐
34.	The breasts are accessory organs to the female reproductive system	True ☐ False ☐
35.	An ectopic pregnancy is a pregnancy that occurs inside the uterus	True ☐ False ☐
36.	The penis carries urine from the urethra	True ☐ False ☐
37.	The perineum is the skin between the vagina and the anus	True ☐ False ☐

38.	The mons pubis protects the entrance to the vagina	True ☐ False ☐
39.	From month 4 the gender of the foetus is recognisable	True ☐ False ☐
40.	The breasts are supported by coopers ligaments	True ☐ False ☐

Exercise 2

Complete the following crossword on The Reproductive System by answering the clues below.

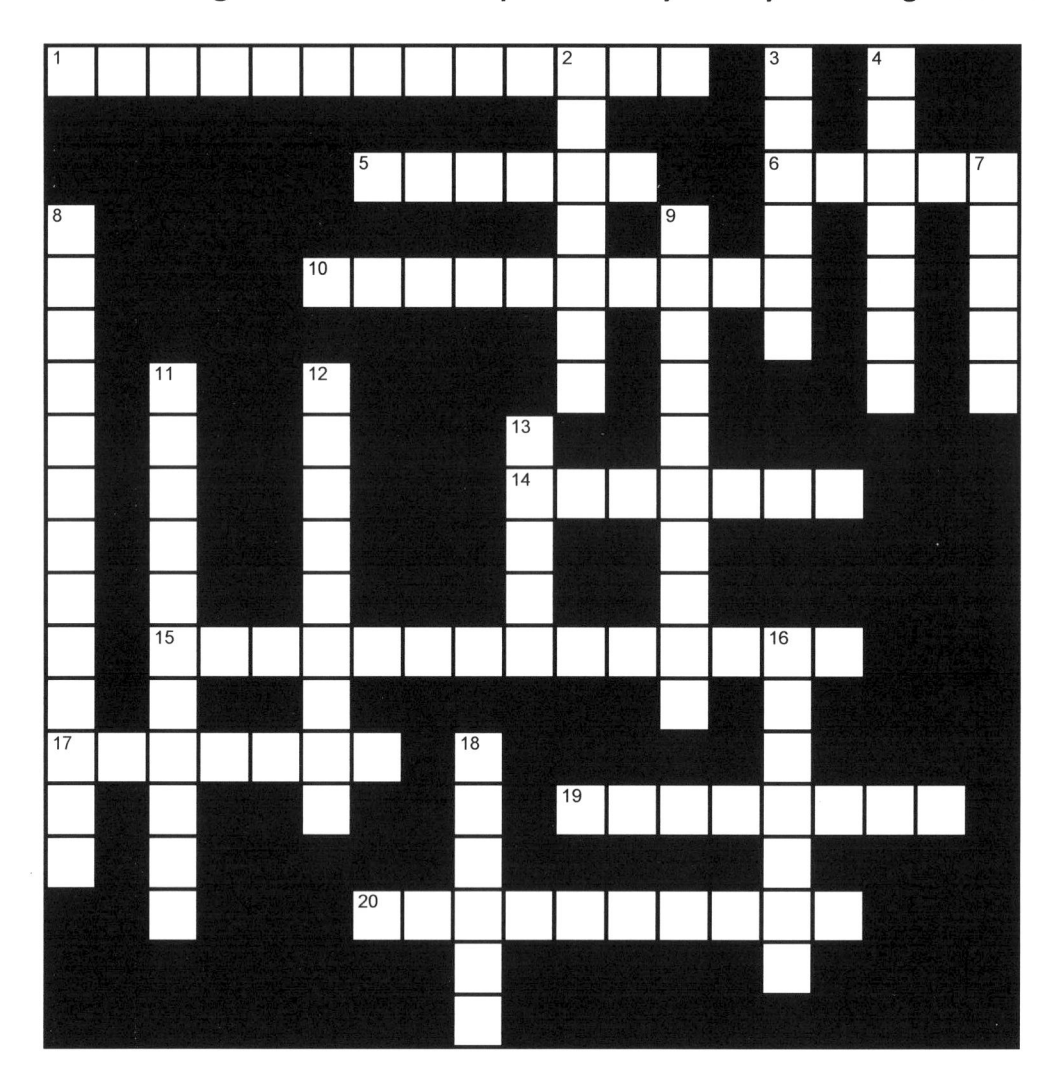

Across

1. What part of the male reproductive system secretes a thin, milky fluid that forms part of the seminal fluid? (13)
5. What part of the uterus dilates during childbirth to allow the passage of the baby? (6)
6. The tip of the penis (5)
10. What develops from the zygote 5 days after fertilisation? (10)
14. What tube runs through centre of the penis providing a pathway for urine and semen? (7)
15. What part of the female reproductive system carries the ovum from ovaries to uterus? (14)
17. What supports and protects the testes? (7)
19. What is protected by the labia minora? (8)
20. Where are immature sperm cells stored? (10)

Down

2. What type of connective tissue are the breasts mainly made up of? (7)
3. What cell is formed after the sperm fertilises an egg? (6)
4. What glands secrete female hormones? (7)
7. What fertilises the ovum? (5)
8. What is the condition called where the tissue that normally lines the uterus grows on other organs outside the uterus? (13)
9. What is the middle layer of the uterus wall called? (10)
11. What tube leads from the epididymis to the urethra? (11)
12. What creates movement in the sperm enabling it to propel towards the ovum? (9)
13. What are the external sexual organs of the female reproductive system called? (5)
16. What type of pregnancy occurs outside the uterus? (7)
18. What connects the internal and external sex organs of the female reproductive system? (6)

Exercise3

In the table below, match what parts of the reproductive system belong to either the Male or Female Reproductive Systems.

1.	Ovaries		11.	Scrotum	
2.	Prostate Gland		12.	Labia Majora	
3.	Epididymis		13.	Graafian Follicle	
4.	Labia Minora		14.	Penis	
5.	Testes		15.	Fallopian Tubes	
6.	Cervix		16.	Clitoris	
7.	Mons Pubis		17.	Glans	
8.	Vas Deferens		18.	Uterus	
9.	Mammary Glands		19.	Sperm	
10.	Vagina		20.	Flagellum	

Exercise 4

Please answer the questions below and find the answers in the word search puzzle.

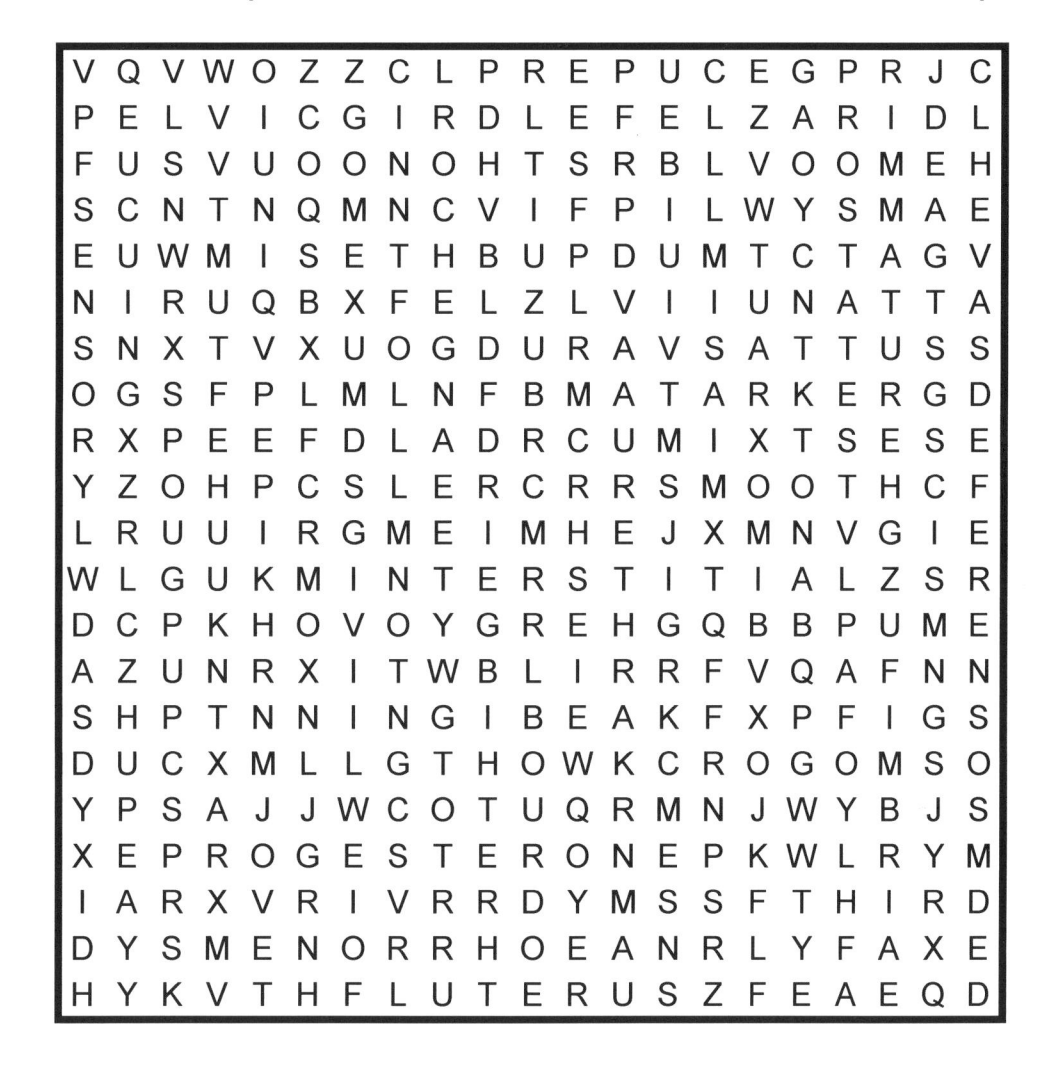

```
V Q V W O Z Z C L P R E P U C E G P R J C
P E L V I C G I R D L E F E L Z A R I D L
F U S V U O O N O H T S R B L V O O M E H
S C N T N Q M N C V I F P I L W Y S M A E
E U W M I S E T H B U P D U M T C T A G V
N I R U Q B X F E L Z L V I I U N A T T A
S N X T V X U O G D U R A V S A T T U S S
O G S F P L M L N F B M A T A R K E R G D
R X P E E F D L A D R C U M I X T S E S E
Y Z O H P C S L E R C R R S M O O T H C F
L R U U I R G M E I M H E J X M N V G I E
W L G U K M I N T E R S T I T I A L Z S R
D C P K H O V O Y G R E H G Q B B P U M E
A Z U N R X I T W B L I R R F V Q A F N N
S H P T N N I N G I B E A K F X P F I G S
D U C X M L L G T H O W K C R O G O M S O
Y P S A J J W C O T U Q R M N J W Y B J S
X E P R O G E S T E R O N E P K W L R Y M
I A R X V R I V R R D Y M S S F T H I R D
D Y S M E N O R R H O E A N R L Y F A X E
H Y K V T H F L U T E R U S Z F E A E Q D
```

1. What protects the male and female internal sex organs? (12)
2. A walnut size male accessory gland positioned between the bladder and the rectum (8)
3. What type of sperm are stored and developed in the epididymis? (8)
4. What glands secrete mucus, helping to lubricate the vulva? (10)
5. What type of muscle tissue makes up the myometrium? (6)
6. What type of nerve endings are found around the nipples? (7)
7. What group of cells in the testes produce the male sex hormones? (12)
8. What hormone increases blood flow to the breasts during the menstrual cycle? (12)
9. Where does the embryo grow and develop? (6)
10. What are the finger-like projections found at the end of fallopian tubes called? (8)
11. What part of the male reproductive system is cut during a vasectomy? (11)
12. What is very painful menstruation known as? (13)
13. What type of tissue is the penis composed of? (8)

Anatomy & Physiology Student Workbook

14. During what month of pregnancy do the teeth begin to develop? (5)
15. Term used to describe the external genitalia in the female reproductive system (5)
16. What skin surrounds and protects the glans? (7)
17. What is the process called when an ovum is released every month? (9)
18. Where does the foetus grow and develop within the uterus? (14)
19. What occurs in a woman when the menstrual cycle ends? (9)
20. What provides a passageway for urine and semen? (7)

Exercise 5

Fill in the missing words

1. The testes are the _____ glands of the male system (12)

2. During sexual activity the _____ _____ swell from increased blood flow and the penis becomes erect (5,7)

3. Amenorrhoea is the _____ of menstruation (7)

4. The _____ is the outer layer of the uterus (11)

5. The vas deferens leads from the _____ to the urethra (10)

6. The perimetrium covers the _____ of the uterus (3)

7. An embryo grows and develops into a _____ in the uterus (6)

8. The epididymis stores _____ sperm cells (8)

9. The _____ glands open into the urethra at the base of the penis (7)

10. The fallopian tubes transport ova from the _____ to the uterus (7)

11. The size of the breasts is determined by the amount of _____ tissue (7)

12. The penis is composed of _____ tissue (8)

13. An ectopic pregnancy occurs _____ the uterus (7)

14. Oestrogen is responsible for regulating the development of _____ sexual characteristics (6)

15. The labia _____ protects the entrance to the vagina (6)

Exercise 6

The transport of sperm from the testes to the ovum takes place in 9 stages. Please match those stages in the table below. Stage 1 has been completed.

1.	Testes	**Stage 1**
2.	Fallopian Tubes	
3.	Vas Deferens	
4.	Vagina	
5.	Penis	
6.	Epididymis	
7.	Ovum	
8.	Uterus	
9.	Male Urethra	

Exercise 7

Multiple choice questions, please choose one answer from the 4 choices in each box.

1. How long is the average pregnancy? a) 35 weeks b) 47 weeks c) 40 weeks d) 20 weeks Answer	2. Which one of the following is not a layer of the uterus? a) Endometrium b) Myocardium c) Myometrium d) Perimetrium Answer
3. How many chromosomes does the head of the sperm contain? a) 46 b) 12 c) 23 d) 18 Answer	4. Once the ovum has been fertilised it is known as the; a) Embryo b) Foetus c) Morula d) Zygote Answer
5. What is the function of the ovaries? a) To act as a passageway for sperm b) To fertilise the ovum c) To protect the fertilised ovum d) To produce the ovum Answer	6. What protects the uterus? a) Pelvis b) Ribs c) Abdominal wall d) Cervix Answer
7. What is responsible for supplying the developing baby with oxygen and nutrients? a) Placenta b) Blastocyst c) Amniotic cavity d) Embryo Answer	8. What extends from the top of the uterus ending near each ovary? a) Fimbriae b) Uterus c) Fallopian tubes d) Urethra Answer

9. What are the male reproductive glands? a) Epididymis b) Sperm c) Cowper's glands d) Testes Answer	10. The absence of menstruation is known as; a) Dysmenorrhoea b) Polycystic Ovarian Syndrome c) Endometriosis d) Amenorrhoea Answer
11. What is the tip of the penis called? a) Prepuce b) Glans c) Flagellum d) Foreskin Answer	12. What is the term used to describe giving birth? a) Defecation b) Micturition c) Parturition d) Pronation Answer
13. Which one of the following is not part of the vulva? a) Cervix b) Labia minora c) Mons pubis d) Clitoris Answer	14. Where does sperm have to travel to, to reach the ovum? a) Uterus b) Vagina c) Ovaries d) Fallopian tubes Answer
15. Where are the testes held? a) Testicular vessels b) Scrotum c) Penis d) Prostate gland Answer	16. Why is sperm stored in the testes? a) It needs to be kept at a lower temperature than the body b) It needs to develop and mature before being carried to the prostate gland c) It needs to receive further secretions from the prostate gland d) It needs to be kept at the normal body temperature Answer

17. What determines when childbirth should begin? a) The length of the perineum b) The dilation of the vagina c) The dilation of the cervix d) The birth of the placenta Answer	**18. What is the function of the vas deferens?** a) To store sperm b) To transport sperm from the epididymis to the urethra c) To secrete part of the seminal fluids d) To protect and support the testes Answer
19. What type of tissue is found in the breasts? a) Adipose b) Yellow elastic c) Nervous d) Hyaline Answer	**20. How long after fertilisation is the embryo known as the foetus?** a) 24 days b) 10 weeks c) 8 weeks d) 5 days Answer
21. What is found on the surface of each ovary? a) Follicles b) Glands c) Tissue d) Tubes Answer	**22. What runs down the centre of the penis?** a) Glans b) Erectile tissue c) Urethra d) Prepuce Answer
23. Where is the prostate gland positioned? a) Between the bladder and rectum b) Between the perineum and the anus c) Between the bladder and scrotum d) Between the kidneys Answer	**24. What is the mass of cells produced from the zygote called?** a) Embryo b) Bolus c) Blastocyst d) Morula Answer

25. What part of the sperm contains the nucleus?	**26. Why is the pelvic girdle wider in women?**
a) Flagellum	a) To support the uterus
b) Head	b) To allow room for a baby to be born
c) Tail	c) Because the female sex organs are internal
d) Chromosomes	d) To protect the female reproductive organs
Answer _____	Answer _____
27. What is the function of Cowper's glands?	**28. Inflammation of the prostate gland is known as;**
a) To supply the penis with blood vessels	a) Endometriosis
b) To allow for the passage of sperm from the urethra to the penis	b) Dysmenorrhoea
c) To produce mucus, lubricating the urethra	c) Prostatitis
d) To produce secretions for seminal fluid	d) Fibrodosis
Answer _____	Answer _____
29. When is the gender of the foetus distinguishable?	**30. What is the areola?**
a) At the end of the 3rd trimester	a) The tissue that makes up the breast
b) At the beginning of the 2nd trimester	b) The skin around the nipple
c) At the end of the 4th trimester	c) The ducts that support breast tissue
d) At the end of the 2nd trimester	d) The muscle behind the breast
Answer _____	Answer _____
31. Which one of the following is not part of the male reproductive system?	**32. What is an immature ova called?**
a) Glans	a) Oocytes
b) Fimbriae	b) Ovum
c) Flagellum	c) Eggs
d) Vas deferens	d) Zygotes
Answer _____	Answer _____

33. What type of epithelium is found in the fallopian tubes? a) Ciliated b) Columnar c) Squamous d) Cuboidal Answer	**34. What is another name for foreskin?** a) Glans b) Nucleus c) Prepuce d) Semen Answer
35. What is the fluid discharged from the penis during intercourse? a) Sperm b) Mucus c) Amniotic fluid d) Semen Answer	**36. Which one of the following is not part of the penis?** a) Erectile tissue b) Lymphatic vessels c) Urethra d) Prepuce Answer
37. Which one of the following is the fluid filled sac that contains the embryo? a) Uterus b) Mons pubis c) Amniotic cavity d) Foetus Answer	**38. What part of the vulva protects the entrance to the vagina?** a) Labia minora b) Mons pubis c) Labia majora d) Clitoris Answer
39. What tube runs from each testis to the vas deferens? a) Prostate gland b) Seminal vesicle c) Urethra d) Epididymis Answer	**40. How many sperm are needed to fertilise an ovum?** a) 1 million b) 1 c) 10 d) 1 thousand Answer

Anatomy & Physiology Student Workbook

The Reproductive System

Answers

Exercise 1 (true/false):

1. False	11. False	21. False	31. True
2. True	12. True	22. False	32. True
3. False	13. False	23. True	33. False
4. False	14. True	24. False	34. True
5. True	15. True	25. False	35. False
6. True	16. True	26. True	36. False
7. True	17. False	27. True	37. True
8. False	18. False	28. False	38. False
9. True	19. True	29. True	39. True
10. False	20. True	30. False	40. True

Exercise 2 (crossword):

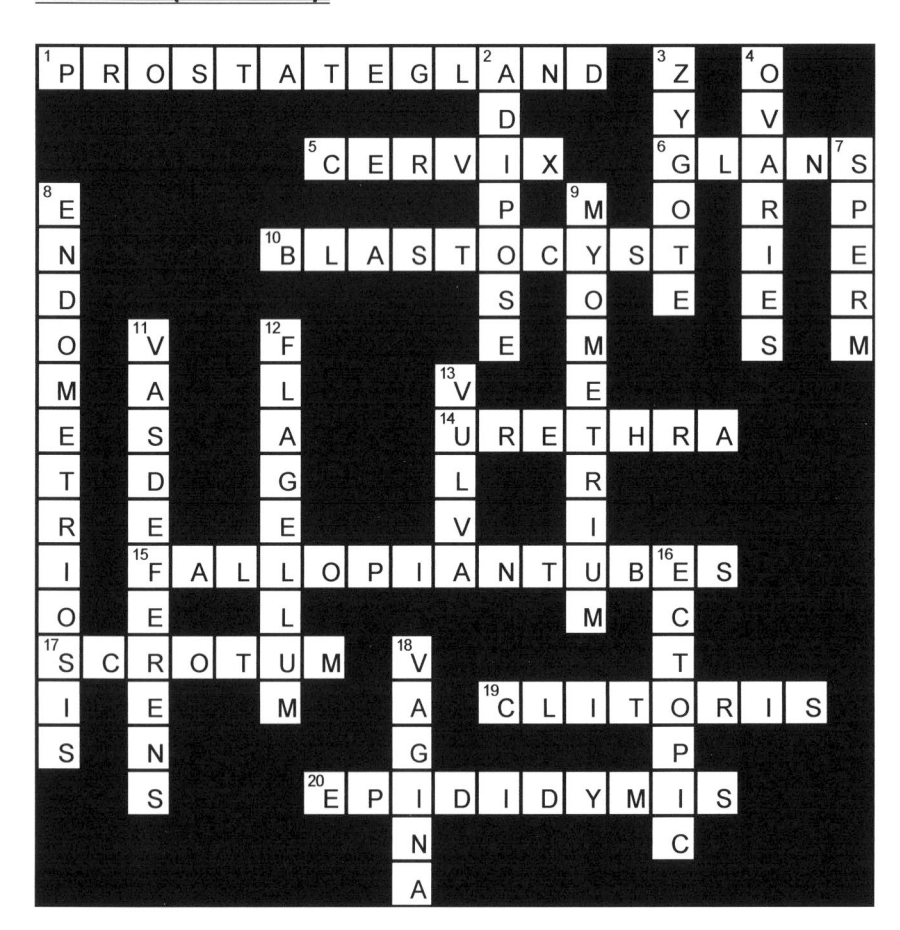

1 Across: PROSTATEGLAND
2 Down: ADDS (ADD...)
3 Down: ZY...
4 Down: OV...
5 Across: CERVIX
6 Across: GLANS
7 Down: SPERM...
8 Down: ENDOMETRIUM
9 Down: MO...
10 Across: BLASTOCYST
11 Down: VAS DEFERENS
12 Down: FLAGELLE
13 Down: VULV...
14 Across: URETHRA
15 Across: FALLOPIAN TUBES
16 Down: ESCT...
17 Across: SCROTUM
18 Down: VAGINA
19 Across: CLITORIS
20 Across: EPIDIDYMIS

Anatomy & Physiology Student Workbook — Page 214

Exercise 3 (match what parts of the reproductive systems belong to either the male or female systems):

1. Female
2. Male
3. Male
4. Female
5. Male
6. Female
7. Female
8. Male
9. Female
10. Female
11. Male
12. Female
13. Female
14. Male
15. Female
16. Female
17. Male
18. Female
19. Male
20. Male

Exercise 4 (word search):

1. Pelvic Girdle
2. Prostate
3. Immature
4. Vestibular
5. Smooth
6. Sensory
7. Interstitial
8. Progesterone
9. Uterus
10. Fimbriae
11. Vas Deferens
12. Dysmenorrhoea
13. Erectile
14. Third
15. Vulva
16. Prepuce
17. Ovulation
18. Amniotic Cavity
19. Menopause
20. Urethra

Exercise 5 (fill in the missing words):

1. Reproductive
2. Blood Vessels
3. Absence
4. Perimetrium
5. Epididymis
6. Top
7. Foetus
8. Immature
9. Cowpers
10. Ovaries
11. Adipose
12. Erectile
13. Outside
14. Female
15. Majora

Anatomy & Physiology Student Workbook

Exercise 6 (the transport of sperm from the testes to the ovum takes place in 9 stages, match these stages):

1. Stage 1
2. Stage 8
3. Stage 3
4. Stage 6
5. Stage 5
6. Stage 2
7. Stage 9
8. Stage 7
9. Stage 4

Exercise 7 (multiple choice questions):

1	C	9	D	17	C	25	B	33	A
2	B	10	D	18	B	26	B	34	C
3	C	11	B	19	A	27	D	35	D
4	D	12	C	20	C	28	C	36	B
5	D	13	A	21	A	29	A	37	C
6	A	14	D	22	C	30	B	38	C
7	A	15	B	23	A	31	B	39	D
8	C	16	A	24	D	32	A	40	B

Chapter 10 | The Respiratory System

Revision Puzzles & Questions

Exercise 1

The following grid lists statements on the left that are either true or false. Please choose your answer on the right. All answers are provided at the end of the chapter.

1.	The lungs are the main muscles of respiration	True ☐ False ☐
2.	During exhalation the diaphragm contracts and flattens out	True ☐ False ☐
3.	Air travels from the larynx to the trachea	True ☐ False ☐
4.	The pharynx is a large tube made of adipose tissue	True ☐ False ☐
5.	The larynx is also known as the voice box	True ☐ False ☐
6.	The lungs are positioned in the thoracic cavity	True ☐ False ☐
7.	Pleurisy describes inflammation of the lungs	True ☐ False ☐

8.	External respiration is an involuntary movement controlled by the hypothalamus	True ☐ False ☐
9.	The bronchi connect the trachea to the lungs	True ☐ False ☐
10.	Dermal papillae are tiny hairs found in the nose which help to move the mucus into the throat	True ☐ False ☐
11.	Alveoli are made of squamous epithelial cells	True ☐ False ☐
12.	Inspiration occurs when we breath in air	True ☐ False ☐
13.	During inhalation the external intercostals muscles help to lift the rib cage down and inwards	True ☐ False ☐
14.	Inflammation of the bronchial tubes is known as bronchitis	True ☐ False ☐
15.	The respiratory centre is controlled by the medulla oblongata	True ☐ False ☐
16.	The larynx connects the trachea to the bronchi	True ☐ False ☐
17.	The pleura is a membrane surrounding the lungs	True ☐ False ☐

18.	Air in the nose is moistened by mucus	True ☐ False ☐
19.	Carbon dioxide is released into the air that is breathed out of the alveoli	True ☐ False ☐
20.	The alveoli are the final passageways of air to the lungs	True ☐ False ☐
21.	The inner layer of the pleura is known as the parietal layer	True ☐ False ☐
22.	The trachea is made up of yellow elastic cartilage	True ☐ False ☐
23.	Air travels from the bronchioles to the alveoli of the lungs	True ☐ False ☐
24.	Emphysema occurs when the alveoli become stretched and damaged	True ☐ False ☐
25.	When the diaphragm relaxes it flattens out	True ☐ False ☐
26.	The intercostal muscles are positioned between the ribs	True ☐ False ☐
27.	The tonsils are found at the back of the larynx	True ☐ False ☐

28.	The trachea is made up of smooth muscle	True ☐ False ☐
29.	Internal respiration is when the oxygen diffuses from the blood into the body's cells	True ☐ False ☐
30.	The bronchi are made up of voluntary muscle	True ☐ False ☐
31.	The exchange of gases takes place in the alveoli of the lungs	True ☐ False ☐
32.	The visceral layer is attached to the surface of the lungs	True ☐ False ☐
33.	Systemic circulation involves the transport of blood from the heart to the lungs	True ☐ False ☐
34.	Inflammation of the pharynx is known as pharyngitis	True ☐ False ☐
35.	The pharynx divides into the anterior and posterior lobes	True ☐ False ☐
36.	Elastic tissue can be found in bronchioles	True ☐ False ☐
37.	The pleural cavity separates the visceral and parietal layers	True ☐ False ☐

38.	The blood collects the oxygen in the cells and brings it to the lungs where it is exchanged for carbon dioxide	True ☐ False ☐
39.	The trachea is lined with ciliated epithelium	True ☐ False ☐
40.	Nerve cells called neurotransmitters send impulses to the medulla oblongata with messages about oxygen and carbon dioxide levels in the blood	True ☐ False ☐

Exercise 2

The passage of air throughout the respiratory system goes through 9 stages. Please match the stages in the table below. Stage 1 has been completed for you.

1.	Nose	Stage 1
2.	Larynx	
3.	Bronchi	
4.	Nasopharynx	
5.	Lungs	
6.	Trachea	
7.	Pharynx	
8.	Alveoli	
9.	Bronchioles	

Exercise 3

Complete the following crossword on The Respiratory System by answering the clues below.

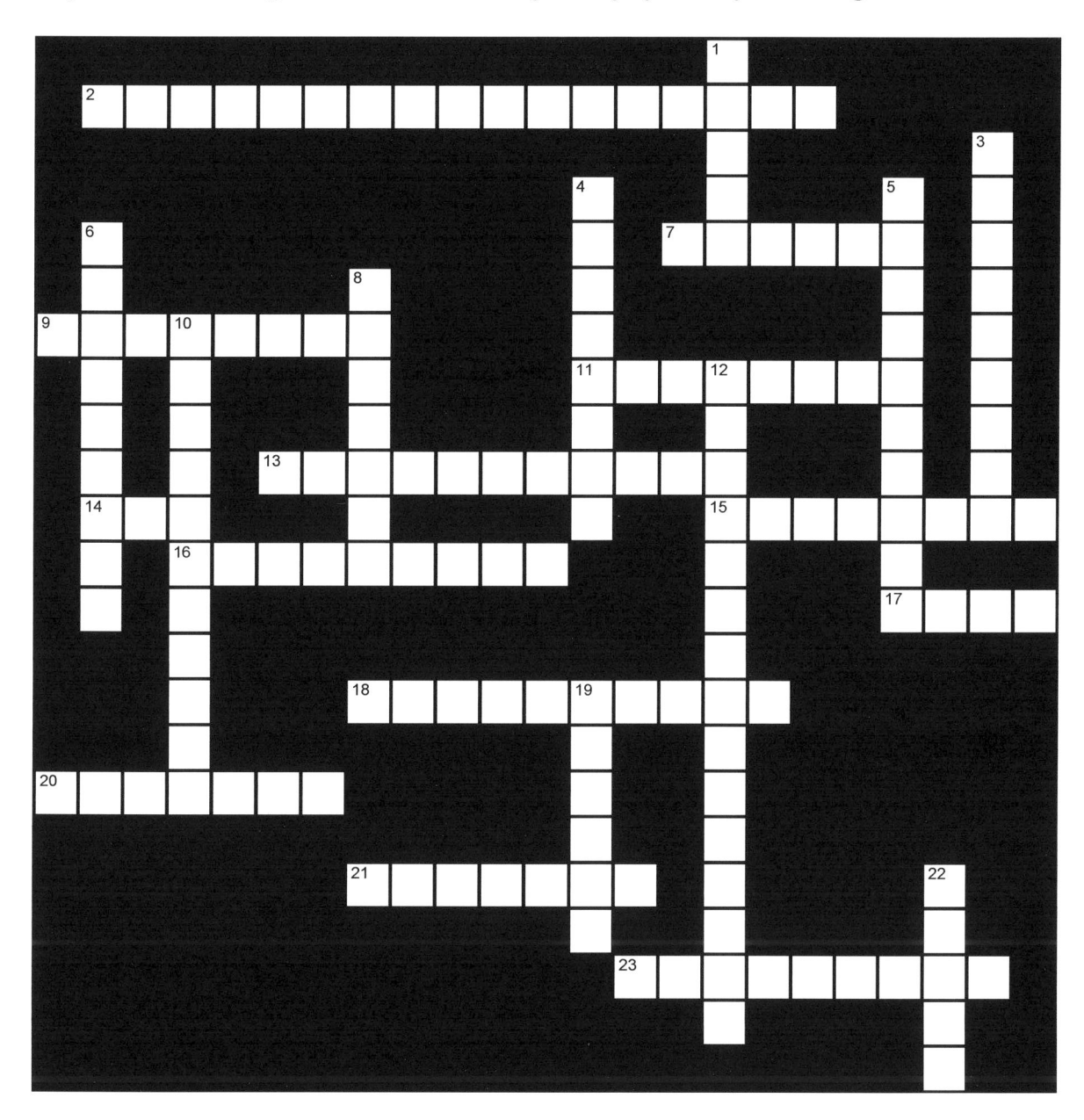

Across
2. What is the cause of a blocked pulmonary artery? (17)
7. What connects the pharynx to the trachea? (6)
9. What layer of the pleura lines the thoracic cavity? (8)
11. What type of respiration occurs when carbon dioxide diffuses from the blood into the air inside the alveoli? (8)
13. The alveoli receive air from what part of the respiratory system? (11)
14. What passes through the pharynx into the larynx? (3)

15. What are the end of bronchioles called? (8)
16. What tissue is found inside the larynx? (9)
17. What is the organ of smell? (4)
18. What tissue, found in the larynx, prevents food from going down the wrong way? (10)
20. What type of cartilage is the bronchi composed of? (7)
21. What part of the respiratory system is made up of rings of cartilage? (7)
23. What is the term used to describe the inhalation and exhalation of air? (9)

Down
1. What filters the incoming air in the nose? (5)
3. Inflammation of the lungs (9)
4. What is another name for the larynx? (8)
5. What occurs when the diaphragm relaxes and the chest cavity narrows? (10)
6. What muscle is positioned between the thoracic cavity and the abdomen? (9)
8. What part of the respiratory system is made up of squamous epithelial cells and very small capillaries? (7)
10. What group of muscles help the diaphragm in respiration? (11)
12. What opens into the nasopharynx balancing the air pressure inside the ear? (15)
19. What is diffused from the blood into the body's cells during internal respiration? (6)
22. What organs are positioned either side of the heart? (5)

Exercise 4

Fill in the missing words.

1. The bronchi connect the _____ to the lungs (7)

2. Expiration occurs when the diaphragm _____ (7)

3. Bronchioles become smaller and divide into _____ bronchioles (8)

4. During external respiration _____ diffuses from the alveoli into the bloodstream (6)

5. The nose is the organ of _____ (5)

6. When air passes over the _____ _____ in the larynx it produces sound (5,5)

7. The respiratory and _____ systems work very closely together during the exchange of gases in the lungs (11)

8. During external respiration carbon dioxide is transported by the blood from the cells of the body to the _____ surrounding the alveoli (11)

9. Pleurisy occurs due to _____ of the pleura lining (12)

10. The trachea is made up of _____ muscle (6)

11. The air is _____ in the nose by cilia (8)

12. Air travels from the nose to the nasopharynx, on to the _____ and is then received by the larynx (7)

13. The _____ sinuses open into the nasal cavity (9)

14. The volume of the chest cavity is _____ during exhaling (9)

15. The medulla oblongata is responsible for controlling the _____ centre (11)

Exercise 5

Please answer the questions below and find the answers in the word search puzzle.

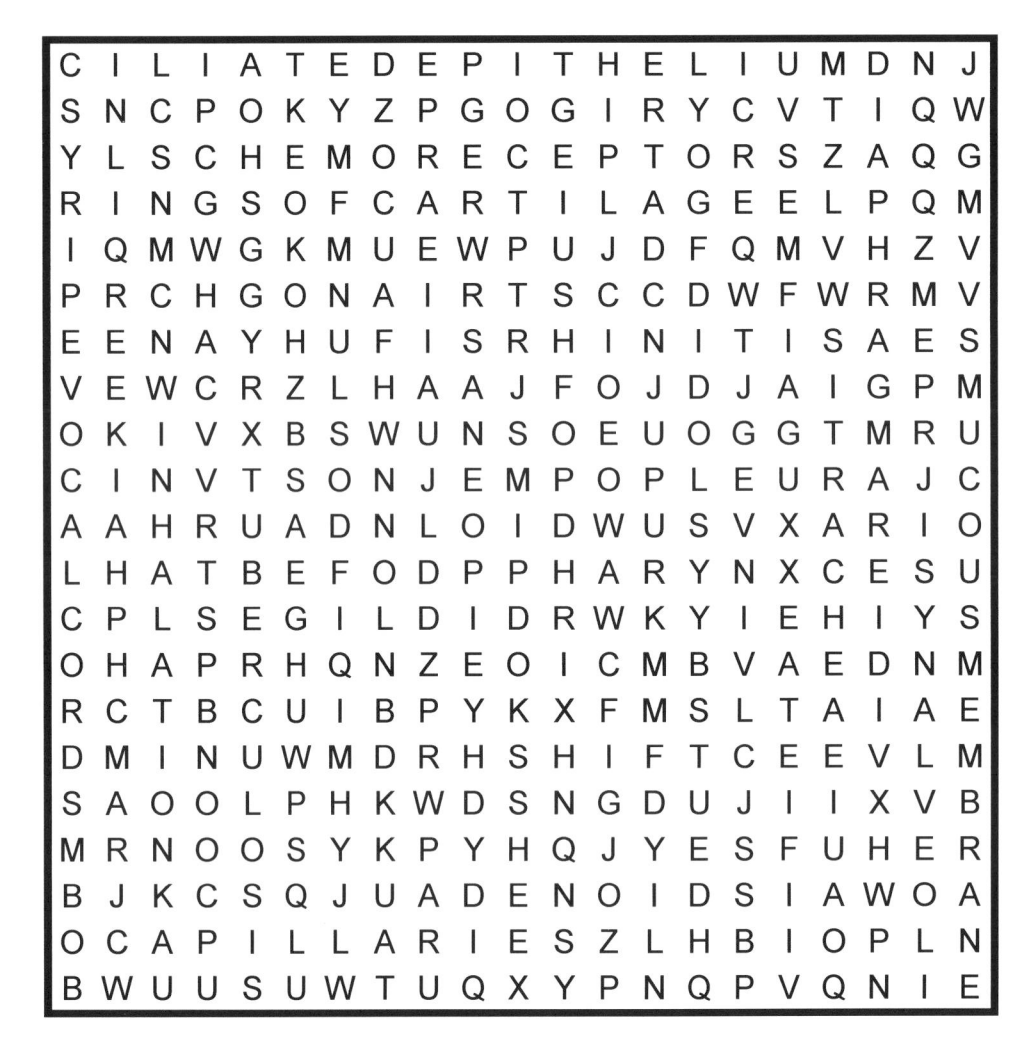

```
C I L I A T E D E P I T H E L I U M D N J
S N C P O K Y Z P G O G I R Y C V T I Q W
Y L S C H E M O R E C E P T O R S Z A Q G
R I N G S O F C A R T I L A G E E L P Q M
I Q M W G K M U E W P U J D F Q M V H Z V
P R C H G O N A I R T S C C D W F W R M V
E E N A Y H U F I S R H I N I T I S A E S
V E W C R Z L H A A J F O J D J A I G P M
O K I V X B S W U N S O E U O G G T M R U
C I N V T S O N J E M P O P L E U R A J C
A A H R U A D N L O I D W U S V X A R I O
L H A T B E F O D P P H A R Y N X C E S U
C P L S E G I L D I D R W K Y I E H I Y S
O H A P R H Q N Z E O I C M B V A E D N M
R C T B C U I B P Y K X F M S L T A I A E
D M I N U W M D R H S H I F T C E E V L M
S A O O L P H K W D S N G D U J I I X V B
M R N O O S Y K P Y H Q J Y E S F U H E R
B J K C S Q J U A D E N O I D S I A W O A
O C A P I L L A R I E S Z L H B I O P L N
B W U U S U W T U Q X Y P N Q P V Q N I E
```

1. What substance diffuses from the cells into the blood during internal respiration? (13)
2. What is the trachea also known as? (8)
3. What muscle helps to push up the chest cavity during expiration? (9)
4. In what part of the respiratory system do oxygen and carbon dioxide pass into and out of the bloodstream? (7)
5. What occurs when the diaphragm contracts and flattens out? (10)
6. Inflammation of the mucous membrane of the nose causing a stuffy congested nose (8)
7. What is the bronchi lined with? (18)
8. The tonsils are found at the back of what part of the respiratory system? (7)
9. What can be found in the larynx? (10)
10. What nerve cells send impulses to the medulla oblongata of the brain with messages about oxygen and carbon dioxide levels in the blood? (14)
11. An infectious disease caused by bacteria that commonly affects the lungs (12)
12. What is the process called through which oxygen passes from the alveoli into the blood and

Anatomy & Physiology Student Workbook Page 226

carbon dioxide passes from the blood to the alveoli? (9)
13. What is the nose lined with? (14)
14. What takes air from the bronchi into the alveoli of the lungs? (14)
15. What part of the respiratory system is a passageway for air between larynx and bronchi? (7)
16. What membrane surrounds each lung? (6)
17. What type of blood vessels surround the alveoli to help with the exchange of gases? (11)
18. What enables the trachea to hold its shape? (16)
19. What groups of lymphoid tissue are located at the back of the nasopharynx? (8)

Exercise 6

In the table below, please match whether the actions within the chest relate to <u>inhalation or exhalation</u>.

1.	The diaphragm relaxes	
2.	Thoracic cavity pushes up	
3.	Pressure inside the chest is lowered	
4.	Diaphragm is a dome shaped	
5.	The thoracic cavity increases in size	
6.	The diaphragm contracts	
7.	The chest cavity decreases in size	
8.	Pressure inside the chest is increased	
9.	The diaphragm flattens out	
10.	The ribs are pulled upwards and outwards	

Exercise 7

Multiple choice questions, please choose one answer from the 4 choices provided in each box.

1. What prevents choking? a) Adrenoids b) Epiglottis c) Cilia d) Tonsils Answer	2. What layer of the pleura is attached to the surface of the lungs? a) Parietal b) Pleural cavity c) Ciliated cells d) Visceral Answer
3. What part of the brain is responsible for controlling most of the respiratory system's functions? a) Hypothalamus b) Midbrain c) Cerebrum d) Medulla oblongata Answer	4. What connects the larynx to the bronchi? a) Pharynx b) Bronchioles c) Trachea d) Nose Answer
5. What disorder of the respiratory system occurs when the alveoli of the lungs become damaged? a) Emphysema b) Pneumonia c) Tuberculosis d) Pleurisy Answer	6. What type of connective tissue are the adenoids composed of? a) Lymphoid b) Areolar c) Yellow elastic d) Adipose Answer
7. What is the main muscle of respiration? a) External intercostals b) Rectus abdominis c) Diaphragm d) Pectoralis major Answer	8. Which one of the following is not a function of the respiratory system? a) Enables smell b) Produces enzymes c) Produces speech d) Exchanges gases in and out of the lungs Answer

9. Which one of the following does not contain cartilage?
a) Bronchioles
b) Trachea
c) Larynx
d) Bronchi

Answer
_____

10. What type of membrane is the nose lined with?
a) Fibrous
b) Serous
c) Mucous
d) Fluid

Answer
_____

11. The windpipe is a common name for the;
a) Bronchi
b) Pharynx
c) Larynx
d) Trachea

Answer
_____

12. What passes over the vocal cords enabling sound?
a) Gas
b) Hydrogen
c) Carbon dioxide
d) Air

Answer
_____

13. Inspiration occurs;
a) When the diaphragm contracts
b) When the chest cavity decreases
c) When the chest cavity is pushed up
d) When the diaphragm relaxes

Answer
_____

14. Where is the Adam's Apple formed?
a) Pharynx
b) Larynx
c) Trachea
d) Bronchi

Answer
_____

15. What is the nasal septum made of?
a) Ciliated epithelium
b) Membrane
c) Fibrous tissue
d) Cartilage

Answer
_____

16. What prevents dirt from entering the lungs?
a) Cilia
b) Tissue
c) Trachea
d) Nose

Answer
_____

Anatomy & Physiology Student Workbook

17. What is another term for the voice box?
a) Trachea
b) Windpipe
c) Larynx
d) Pharynx

Answer
_____

18. During external respiration carbon dioxide that is transported from the body's cells is dropped off in the;
a) Bloodstream
b) Capillaries
c) Bronchial tubes
d) Lungs

Answer
_____

19. Where in the lungs does the exchange of gases occur?
a) Alveoli
b) Bronchioles
c) Pleura
d) Bronchi

Answer
_____

20. What causes the exchange of gases to take place?
a) Filtration
b) Active transport
c) Osmosis
d) Diffusion

Answer
_____

21. What is another name for the throat?
a) Pharynx
b) Trachea
c) Larynx
d) Bronchi

Answer
_____

22. What is the function of the pleural cavity?
a) To enable a more efficient exchange of gases to take place in the lungs
b) To protect the thoracic cavity which holds the lungs
c) To prevent friction between the visceral and parietal layers
d) To transport air from the trachea into the bronchioles

Answer
_____

23. What enables the sense of smell?
a) Retraction
b) Olfaction
c) Diffusion
d) Inspiration

Answer
_____

24. What is the diffusion of oxygen from the blood into the cells?
a) Pulmonary respiration
b) Internal respiration
c) External respiration
d) Systemic respiration

Answer
_____

25. What is taken from the air that is breathed into the lungs?
a) Carbon dioxide
b) Wastes
c) Bacteria
d) Oxygen

Answer _____

26. During what type of respiration does the blood lose oxygen and gain carbon dioxide?
a) Pulmonary
b) External
c) Diffusion
d) Internal

Answer _____

27. What type of diffusion is responsible for the exchange of gases?
a) Simple
b) Filtered
c) Active
d) Facilitated

Answer _____

28. What is the function of the trachea?
a) To take air from the larynx to the pharynx
b) To take air from the pharynx to the bronchi
c) To take air from the larynx to the bronchi
d) To take air from the pharynx to the larynx

Answer _____

29. Which of the following statements is correct?
a) During exhalation the diaphragm flattens out
b) During inhalation the volume of the chest cavity decreases
c) During exhalation the ribs are pushed up
d) During inhalation the pressure inside the chest cavity is lowered

Answer _____

30. Another term used to describe breathing;
a) Inhalation
b) Internal respiration
c) External respiration
d) Exhalation

Answer _____

31. What is the opening of the larynx called?
a) Hilum
b) Glottis
c) Adenoid
d) Adam's apple

Answer _____

32. What type of epithelial cells are found in the alveoli?
a) Squamous
b) Compound
c) Cuboidal
d) Columnar

Answer _____

33. What is used to prevent tuberculosis? a) Hepatitis B shot b) Antibiotics c) Chemotherapy d) BCG vaccine Answer _____	**34. Where are the intercostal muscles positioned?** a) In the abdominal cavity b) Below the diaphragm c) Between the ribs d) Between the lungs Answer _____
35. What is the outer layer of the pleura called? a) Pleural cavity b) Parietal c) Visceral d) Epiglottis Answer _____	**36. What substance in the nose collects all the dust and stops it from travelling to the lungs?** a) Mucous b) Air c) Dermal papillae d) Sinuses Answer _____
37. What is gaseous exchange? a) The movement of carbon dioxide into the blood and movement of oxygen out of the blood b) The movement of oxygen and carbon dioxide into and out of the cells c) The movement of air into and out of the cells and tissues d) The movement of oxygen out of the alveoli walls Answer _____	**38. What are hollow air pockets found within the bones surrounding the nose?** a) Epiglottis b) Tonsils c) Vacuoles d) Sinuses Answer _____
39. During expiration; a) The ribs are pushed down b) The diaphragm contracts c) The size of the chest cavity increases d) Air is breathed in Answer _____	**40. What occurs when the lungs become solid and fill with fluid?** a) Emphysema b) Bronchitis c) Pneumonia d) Pleurisy Answer _____

The Respiratory System
Answers

Exercise 1 (true/false):

1. False	11. True	21. False	31. True
2. False	12. True	22. False	32. True
3. True	13. False	23. True	33. False
4. False	14. True	24. True	34. True
5. True	15. True	25. False	35. False
6. True	16. False	26. True	36. True
7. False	17. True	27. False	37. True
8. False	18. True	28. True	38. False
9. True	19. True	29. True	39. True
10. False	20. False	30. False	40. False

Exercise 2 (the passage of air goes through 9 stages, match each stage):
1. Stage 1
2. Stage 4
3. Stage 6
4. Stage 2
5. Stage 9
6. Stage 5
7. Stage 3
8. Stage 8
9. Stage 7

Exercise 3 (crossword):

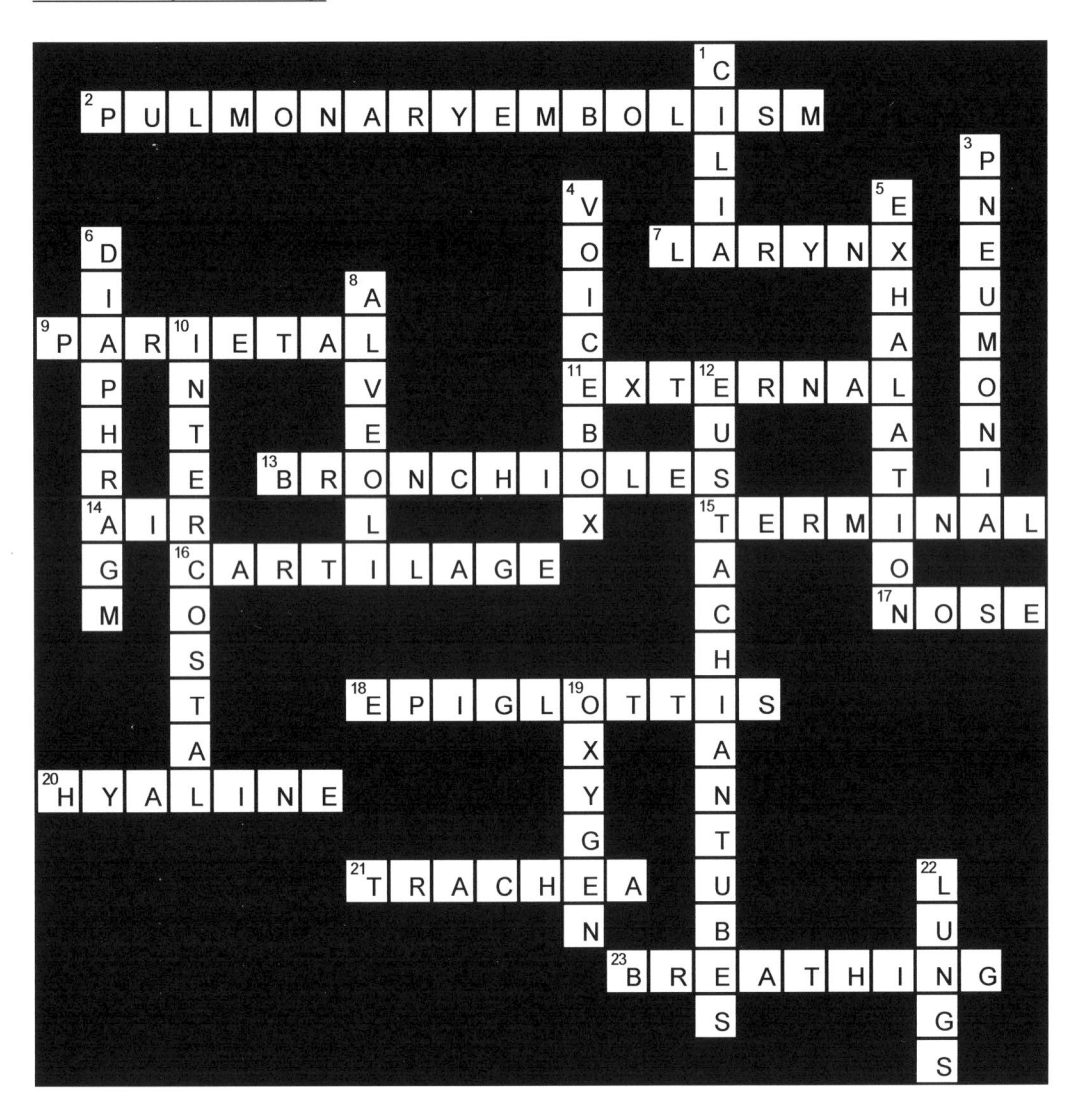

Exercise 4 (fill in the missing words):

1. Trachea
2. Relaxes
3. Terminal
4. Oxygen
5. Smell
6. Vocal Cords
7. Circulatory
8. Capillaries
9. Inflammation
10. Smooth
11. Filtered
12. Pharynx
13. Paranasal
14. Decreased
15. Respiratory

Exercise 5 (word search):

1. Carbon Dioxide
2. Windpipe
3. Diaphragm
4. Alveoli
5. Inhalation
6. Rhinitis
7. Ciliated Epithelium
8. Pharynx
9. Vocal Cords
10. Chemoreceptors
11. Tuberculosis
12. Diffusion
13. Mucous Membrane
14. Bronchioles
15. Trachea
16. Pleura
17. Capillaries
18. Rings of Cartilage
19. Adenoids

Exercise 6 (match whether the actions of the chest are inhalation or exhalation):

1. Exhalation
2. Exhalation
3. Inhalation
4. Exhalation
5. Inhalation
6. Inhalation
7. Exhalation
8. Exhalation
9. Inhalation
10. Inhalation

Exercise 7 (multiple choice questions):

1	B	9	A	17	C	25	D	33	D
2	D	10	C	18	B	26	D	34	C
3	D	11	D	19	A	27	A	35	B
4	C	12	D	20	D	28	C	36	A
5	A	13	A	21	A	29	D	37	B
6	A	14	B	22	C	30	C	38	D
7	C	15	D	23	B	31	B	39	A
8	B	16	A	24	B	32	A	40	C

Anatomy & Physiology Student Workbook

Chapter 11 | The Digestive System

Revision Puzzles & Questions

Exercise 1

The following grid lists statements on the left that are either true or false. Please choose your answer on the right. All answers are provided at the end of the chapter.

1.	The duodenum is part of the large intestine	True ☐ False ☐
2.	The stomach is unable to absorb alcohol	True ☐ False ☐
3.	Rennin curdles milk protein	True ☐ False ☐
4.	Bile is produced in the gall bladder and stored in the liver	True ☐ False ☐
5.	The pancreas, liver and gall bladder are accessory organs to digestion	True ☐ False ☐
6.	Food enters the stomach from the oesophagus via the pyloric sphincter	True ☐ False ☐
7.	Hydrochloric acid neutralises bacteria present in food	True ☐ False ☐

8.	Pepsin is an enzyme found in pancreatic juice	True ☐ False ☐
9.	Vitamins A & D are stored in the liver	True ☐ False ☐
10.	The liver produces heat	True ☐ False ☐
11.	Amylase is involved in fat digestion	True ☐ False ☐
12.	The colon is part of the small intestine	True ☐ False ☐
13.	The oesophagus is the first main organ of digestion	True ☐ False ☐
14.	The oesophagus links the pharynx to the pancreas	True ☐ False ☐
15.	Fat and carbohydrate digestion takes place in the small intestine	True ☐ False ☐
16.	The submandibular gland secretes saliva	True ☐ False ☐
17.	An enzyme is a chemical catalyst which activates chemical changes in itself	True ☐ False ☐

18.	The ball of food at the back of the mouth is known as the bolus	True ☐ False ☐
19.	The peritoneum is a layer of the stomach	True ☐ False ☐
20.	The pancreatic juice, trypsin, breaks down fats into fatty acids and glycerol	True ☐ False ☐
21.	The chemical digestion of food is completed in the small intestine	True ☐ False ☐
22.	Coeliac's disease is caused by an intolerance to a protein called gluten	True ☐ False ☐
23.	Crohn's disease is a disease of the stomach	True ☐ False ☐
24.	The jejunum and ileum are part of the large intestine	True ☐ False ☐
25.	Glucose is an end product of carbohydrate digestion	True ☐ False ☐
26.	The small intestine is 7cm long	True ☐ False ☐
27.	The duodenum is the first part of the small intestine	True ☐ False ☐

28.	Disaccharides and monosaccharides are classified as carbohydrates	True ☐ False ☐
29.	The function of bile is to emulsify proteins	True ☐ False ☐
30.	The liver is the largest gland in the body	True ☐ False ☐
31.	Endocrine and exocrine are functions of the pancreas	True ☐ False ☐
32.	The liver converts stored glycogen to glucose when energy is needed	True ☐ False ☐
33.	Saliva commences the digestion of fats in the mouth	True ☐ False ☐
34.	The pyloric sphincter is located at the entrance to the stomach and prevents the backflow of food from the stomach	True ☐ False ☐
35.	One of the functions of the large intestine is to remove waste	True ☐ False ☐
36.	Iron and potassium are stored by the liver	True ☐ False ☐
37.	Chyme is food broken down into liquid form	True ☐ False ☐

38.	Inflammation of the lining of the stomach is known as enteritis	True ☐ False ☐
39.	Inflammation of the small intestine is known as colitis	True ☐ False ☐
40.	Food remains in the stomach for 2 hours before it becomes chime	True ☐ False ☐

Exercise 2

In the table below, match the digestive organs with the enzymes/fluids they secrete. Choose from the following: 1. Mouth 2. Stomach 3. Duodenum 4. Small Intestine. Some organs may be repeated.

1.	Hydrochloric Acid	
2.	Salivary Amylase	
3.	Lipase	
4.	Rennin	
5.	Maltase	
6.	Trypsin	
7.	Sucrase	
8.	Pepsin	
9.	Amylase	
10.	Lactase	

Exercise 3

Complete the following crossword on The Digestive System by answering the clues below.

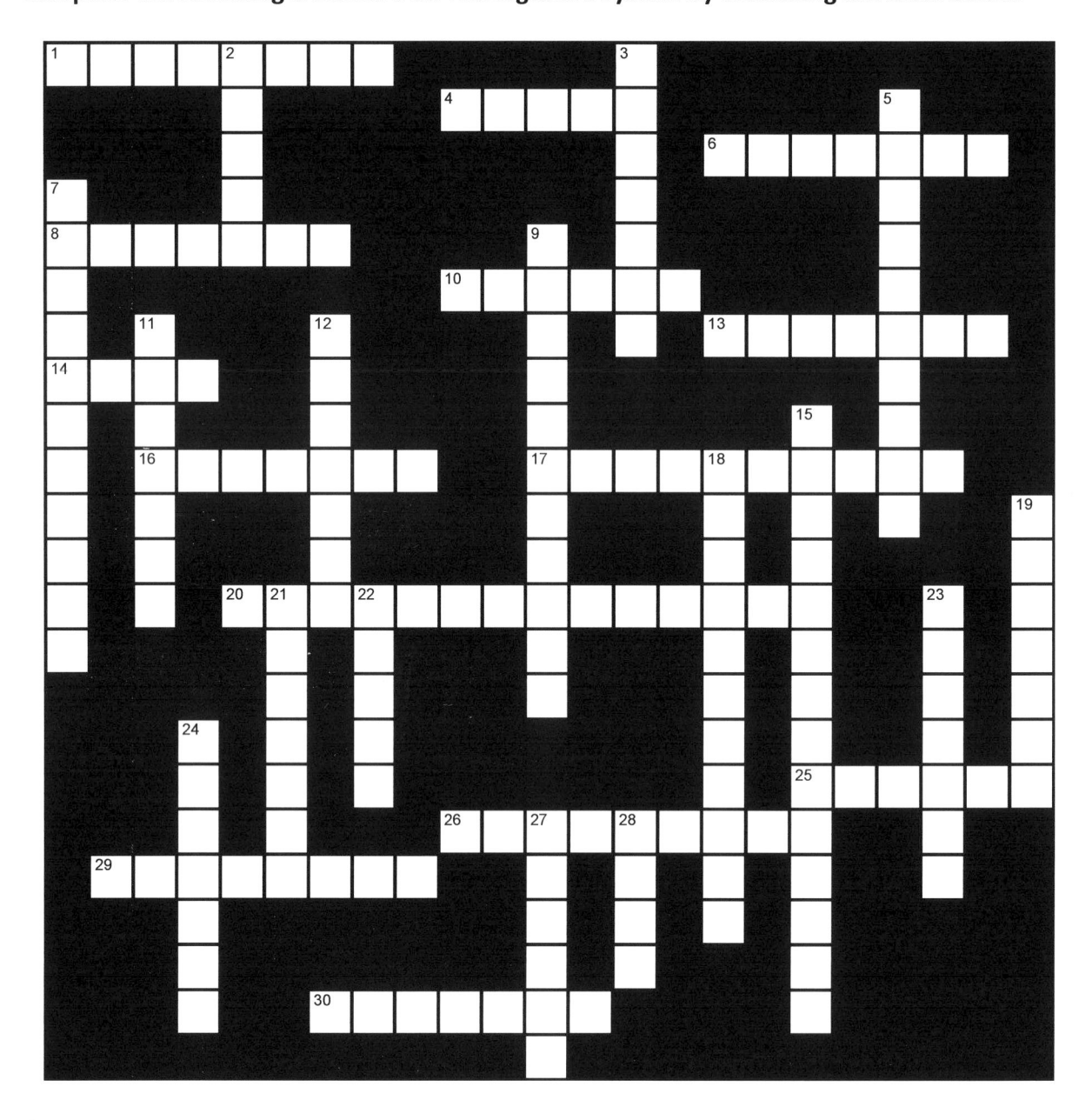

Across
1. What vitamin, essential for maintain healthy teeth and bones, does the liver store? (8)
4. What is food called that has been churned down to a liquid state in the stomach? (5)
6. Pepsin is responsible for commencing the digestion of what food group? (7)
8. What substance does the liver remove? (7)
10. What part of the large intestine does the ileum empty its contents into? (6)
13. What is the last part of the colon called? (7)
14. What alkaline liquid is stored in the gall bladder? (4)

16. What sphincter is responsible for controlling the entry of food into the stomach? (7)
17. What digestive organ receives the bolus from the pharynx? (10)
20. The jejunum belongs to what part of the digestive system? (14)
25. A chemical catalyst (6)
26. A disorder of the digestive system in which liver cells are badly damaged or destroyed (9)
29. The first part of the small intestine (8)
30. Inflammation of the colon (7)

Down
2. Where does the digestion of carbohydrates begin? (5)
3. Part of the small intestine (7)
5. A layer of the stomach that supports the alimentary canal (10)
7. What stores the bile until it is needed? (11)
9. What cells are found inside the liver? (11)
11. What is the end product of carbohydrate digestion? (7)
12. An eating disorder (7)
15. What part of the digestive system is responsible for getting rid of waste? (14)
18. What term is used to describe wave like contractions and relaxations of muscles that occur throughout the digestive tract? (11)
19. An enzyme contained within pancreatic juice (7)
21. What enzyme divides maltose into glucose? (7)
22. What organ stores excess glucose? (5)
23. What pushes the bolus down into the oesophagus? (7)
24. A salivary gland (7)
27. What enzyme coagulates milk in infants? (6)
28. What is produced by the liver? (4)

Exercise 4

Fill in the missing words.

1. The small intestine receives chyme from the _____ (7)

2. Gall stones are formed from changes in the composition of _____ (4)

3. The liver, gall bladder and pancreas are known as _____ organs to digestion (9)

4. The _____ intestine is 1.5 m long (5)

5. Food leaves the stomach through the _____ sphincter and passes into the duodenum (7)

6. The parotid, sublingual and _____ are salivary glands (13)

7. Enzymes are made of _____ (7)

8. The stomach produces _____ which helps to lubricate food (5)

9. Lipase breaks down _____ into fatty acids and glycerol (4)

10. Amylase is involved in _____ digestion (12)

11. _____ is absorbed from the bile in the gall bladder (5)

12. The _____ prevents choking by blocking the entrance to the larynx (10)

13. Sugars and amino acids are absorbed into the walls of the _____ where they pass into the bloodstream (5)

14. The duodenum, the jejunum and the _____ are parts of the small intestine (5)

15. Bile _____ fats (10)

16. Lactase is secreted by the _____ intestine (5)

17. Tiny projections called _____ are found on the surface of the tongue (8)

18. Digestion starts in the _____ (5)

19. The liver converts glycogen into glucose when _____ is needed by the body (6)

20. Pancreatic Juice contains lipase, _____ and trypsin (7)

Exercise 5

Please answer the questions below and find the answers in the word search puzzle.

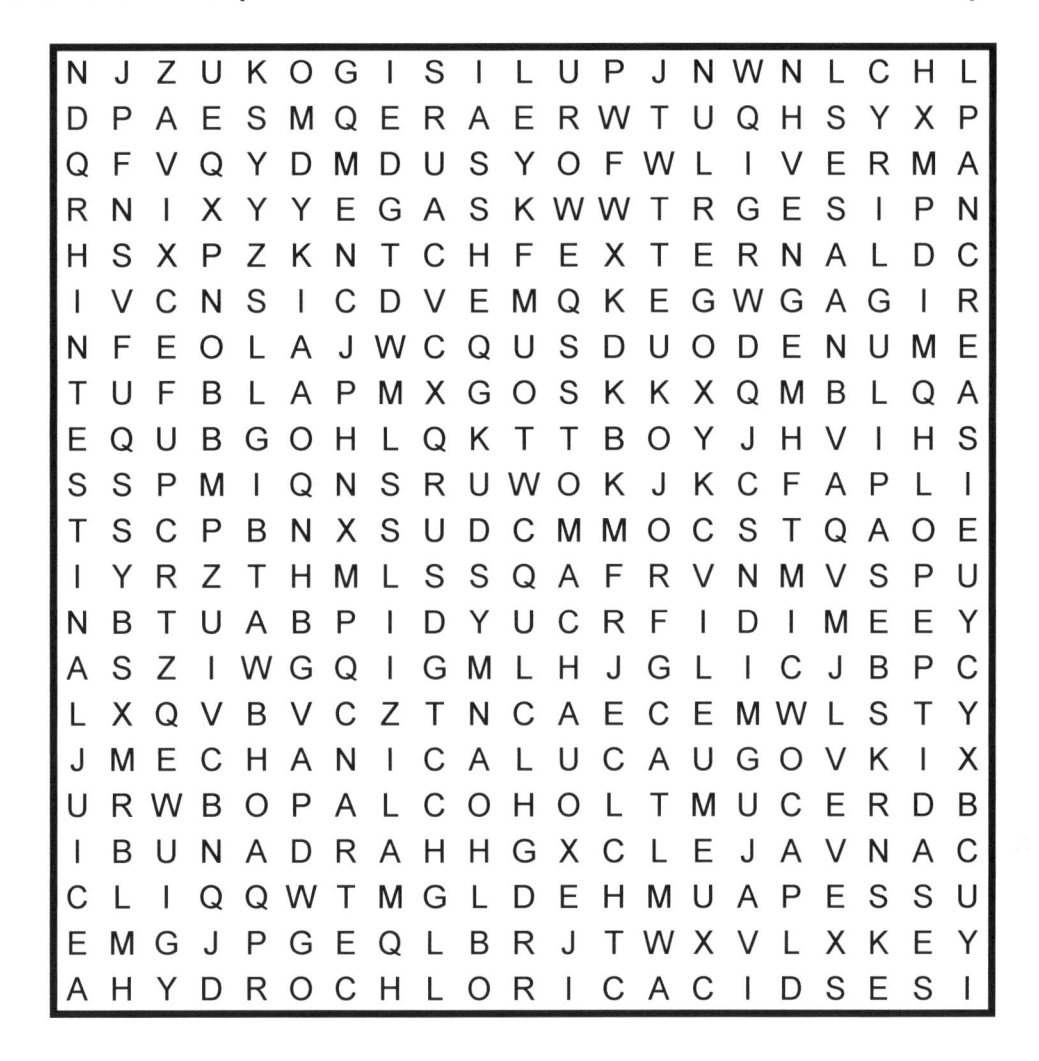

```
N J Z U K O G I S I L U P J N W N L C H L
D P A E S M Q E R A E R W T U Q H S Y X P
Q F V Q Y D M D U S Y O F W L I V E R M A
R N I X Y Y E G A S K W W T R G E S I P N
H S X P Z K N T C H F E X T E R N A L D C
I V C N S I C D V E M Q K E G W G A G I R
N F E O L A J W C Q U S D U O D E N U M E
T U F B L A P M X G O S K K X Q M B L Q A
E Q U B G O H L Q K T T B O Y J H V I H S
S S P M I Q N S R U W O K J K C F A P L I
T S C P B N X S U D C M M O C S T Q A O E
I Y R Z T H M L S S Q A F R V N M V S P U
N B T U A B P I D Y U C R F I D I M E E Y
A S Z I W G Q I G M L H J G L I C J B P C
L X Q V B V C Z T N C A E C E M W L S T Y
J M E C H A N I C A L U C A U G O V K I X
U R W B O P A L C O H O L T M U C E R D B
I B U N A D R A H H G X C L E J A V N A C
C L I Q Q W T M G L D E H M U A P E S S U
E M G J P G E Q L B R J T W X V L X K E Y
A H Y D R O C H L O R I C A C I D S E S I
```

1. Type of digestion involving breaking down solid food into smaller pieces by mastication (10)
2. What are the end products of protein digestion? (10)
3. What part of the large intestine is found between the sigmoid colon and anal canal? (6)
4. What sphincter of the anus is under voluntary control? (8)
5. Where is pancreatic juice produced? (8)
6. What is responsible for chemical reactions during digestion? (7)
7. What is the main section of the large intestine? (5)
8. What substance emulsifies fats? (4)
9. What enzyme converts fats into fatty acids and glycerol? (6)
10. What enzyme helps to complete carbohydrate digestion? (7)
11. A lymph vessel in the small intestine through which fatty acids and glycerol can pass (7)
12. An accessory organ to digestion (5)
13. What enzyme neutralises germs present in food? (16)

Anatomy & Physiology Student Workbook

14. What organ secretes gastric juices? (7)
15. A salivary gland (10)
16. What does the stomach absorb? (7)
17. What organ receives bile from the gall bladder? (8)
18. What is secreted by the small intestine? (15)
19. What splits polypeptides into amino acids? (10)
20. Where does the main absorption of food take place? (5)

Exercise 6

In the table below, match the enzymes of the digestive system with their corresponding functions.

1.	Starts the breakdown of proteins	
2.	Split polypeptides into amino acids	
3.	Kills bacteria present in food	
4.	Split sucrose into glucose and fructose	
5.	End product of carbohydrate digestion	
6.	Starts the digestion of carbohydrates	
7.	End products of fat digestion	
8.	Splits peptones into polypeptides	
9.	Split maltose into glucose	
10.	Split lipids into fatty acids & glycerol	

Please choose from the answers in this box

Lipase	Peptidases	Salivary Amylase	Maltase
Fatty Acids & Glycerol	Sucrase	Trypsin	Hydrochloric Acid
Pepsin	Glucose		

Exercise 7

Multiple choice questions, please choose one answer from the 4 choices provided in each box.

1. What enzyme starts the digestion of proteins in the stomach? a) Pepsin b) Trypsin c) Maltase d) Hydrochloric acid Answer	**2. What is the function of the oesophagus?** a) To carry food from the small intestine to the large intestine b) To carry food from the stomach to the small intestine c) To carry food from the pharynx to the stomach d) To carry food from the mouth to the pharynx Answer
3. What controls the entry of food into the stomach? a) Internal sphincter b) Pyloric sphincter c) External sphincter d) Cardiac sphincter Answer	**4. What is the first organ of digestion?** a) Liver b) Gall bladder c) Oesophagus d) Stomach Answer
5. What is the length of the large intestine? a) 1.5 m b) 7 m c) 8 m d) 2 m Answer	**6. What is the function of lipase?** a) To commence the digestion of protein b) To emulsify fats c) To convert lipids into glycerol and fatty acids d) To convert monosaccharides into disaccharides Answer
7. Where is the pancreas located? a) Above the stomach b) Behind the stomach c) Below the stomach d) In front of the stomach Answer	**8. Which one of the following substances is stored in the liver?** a) Glucose b) Uric acid c) Amino acids d) Iron Answer

9. Which one of the following is not part of the large intestine? a) Caecum b) Ileum c) Appendix d) Colon Answer	**10. What is the function of the gall bladder?** a) To store bile b) To produce heat c) To produce enzymes for digestion d) To metabolise protein Answer
11. What is the main cause of ulcers? a) Excess acid b) Excess bile c) Excess gas d) Excess protein Answer	**12. Crohn's disease occurs in the;** a) Oesophagus b) Duodenum c) Stomach d) Small intestine Answer
13. What enzyme is involved with protein digestion? a) Lipase b) Trypsin c) Amylase d) Bile Answer	**14. What is the function of bile?** a) To convert glycogen into glucose b) To remove toxins from harmful waste c) To convert polypeptides into pepsin d) To emulsify fats Answer
15. Which one of the following vitamins is not stored in the liver? a) Vitamin D b) Vitamin K c) Vitamin E d) Vitamin C Answer	**16. What is enteritis?** a) Inflammation of the pancreas b) Inflammation of the intestine c) Inflammation of the lining of the digestive tract d) Inflammation of the lining of the colon Answer
17. Fats and glycerol pass into; a) Duodenum b) Lacteals c) Blood vessels d) Intestines Answer	**18. What is the order of the sections of the small intestine?** a) Jejunum, ileum, duodenum b) Ileum, duodenum, jejunum c) Duodenum, ileum, jejunum d) Duodenum, jejunum, ileum Answer

19. Amino acids are; a) Proteins b) Carbohydrates c) Vitamins d) Fats Answer	**20. Which one of the following is a type of digestion?** a) Assimilation b) Solid c) Chemical d) Enzyme Answer
21. Where can villi be found? a) Small intestine b) Stomach c) Duodenum d) Pancreas Answer	**22. Where does peristalsis occur?** a) In the larynx b) In the alimentary tract c) In the lungs d) In the gall bladder Answer
23. Which one of the following is not a salivary gland? a) Subtrochlear b) Sublingual c) Parotid d) Submandibular Answer	**24. What is the function of hydrochloric acid?** a) Commences the breakdown of proteins b) Neutralises germs in food c) Curdles milk protein d) Break up large particles of carbohydrates Answer
25. A chemical catalyst; a) A hormone b) An enzyme c) An emulsifier d) A cell Answer	**26. What is the bolus?** a) The enzyme found in the mouth which begins the digestion of carbohydrates b) A chemical catalyst that causes chemical changes in substances c) Where the main absorption of food takes place d) The ball of food that leaves the mouth Answer

27. The chemical digestion of food finishes in the; a) Large intestine b) Stomach c) Small intestine d) Duodenum Answer	**28. What is the length of the small intestine?** a) 3 m b) 1.5 m c) 6 m d) 7 m Answer
29. What is the thick alkaline fluid produced in the liver? a) Glucose b) Amylase c) Bile d) Plasma Answer	**30. What is the largest gland in the body?** a) Liver b) Gall bladder c) Submandibular d) Pancreas Answer
31. What is the term used to describe inflammation of the gums? a) Gall stones b) Appendicitis c) Gingivitis d) Colitis Answer	**32. What part of the alimentary tract is mainly involved with the elimination of waste products?** a) Oesophagus b) Gall bladder c) Pancreas d) Large intestine Answer
33. What type of cells are found in the liver? a) Hepatocytes b) Osteoblasts c) Fibroblasts d) Histioblasts Answer	**34. Which one of the following is not an accessory organ of the digestive system?** a) Liver b) Duodenum c) Gall bladder d) Pancreas Answer

35. What are the end products of protein digestion? a) Glucose b) Fatty acids c) Amino acids d) Glycerol Answer	36. Cirrhosis most commonly affects what organ? a) Liver b) Stomach c) Large intestine d) Pancreas Answer
37. What is the first part of the small intestine? a) Duodenum b) Ileum c) Pancreatic duct d) Jejunum Answer	38. What substance is not found in gastric juice? a) Rennin b) Pepsin c) Trypsin d) Hydrochloric acid Answer
39. Which one of the following enzymes is not involved in the digestion of carbohydrates? a) Maltase b) Lipase c) Lactase d) Sucrase Answer	40. What enzyme begins the digestion of carbohydrates in the mouth? a) Lactase b) Amylase c) Maltase d) Disaccharides Answer

The Digestive System

Answers

Exercise 1 (true/false):

1. False	11. False	21. True	31. True
2. False	12. False	22. True	32. True
3. True	13. True	23. False	33. False
4. False	14. False	24. False	34. False
5. True	15. True	25. True	35. True
6. False	16. True	26. False	36. True
7. True	17. False	27. True	37. True
8. False	18. True	28. True	38. False
9. True	19. True	29. False	39. False
10. True	20. False	30. True	40. False

Exercise 2 (match the digestive organs with the enzymes/fluids they secrete):

1. Stomach
2. Mouth
3. Duodenum
4. Stomach
5. Small Intestine
6. Duodenum
7. Small Intestine
8. Stomach
9. Duodenum
10. Small Intestine

Exercise 3 (crossword):

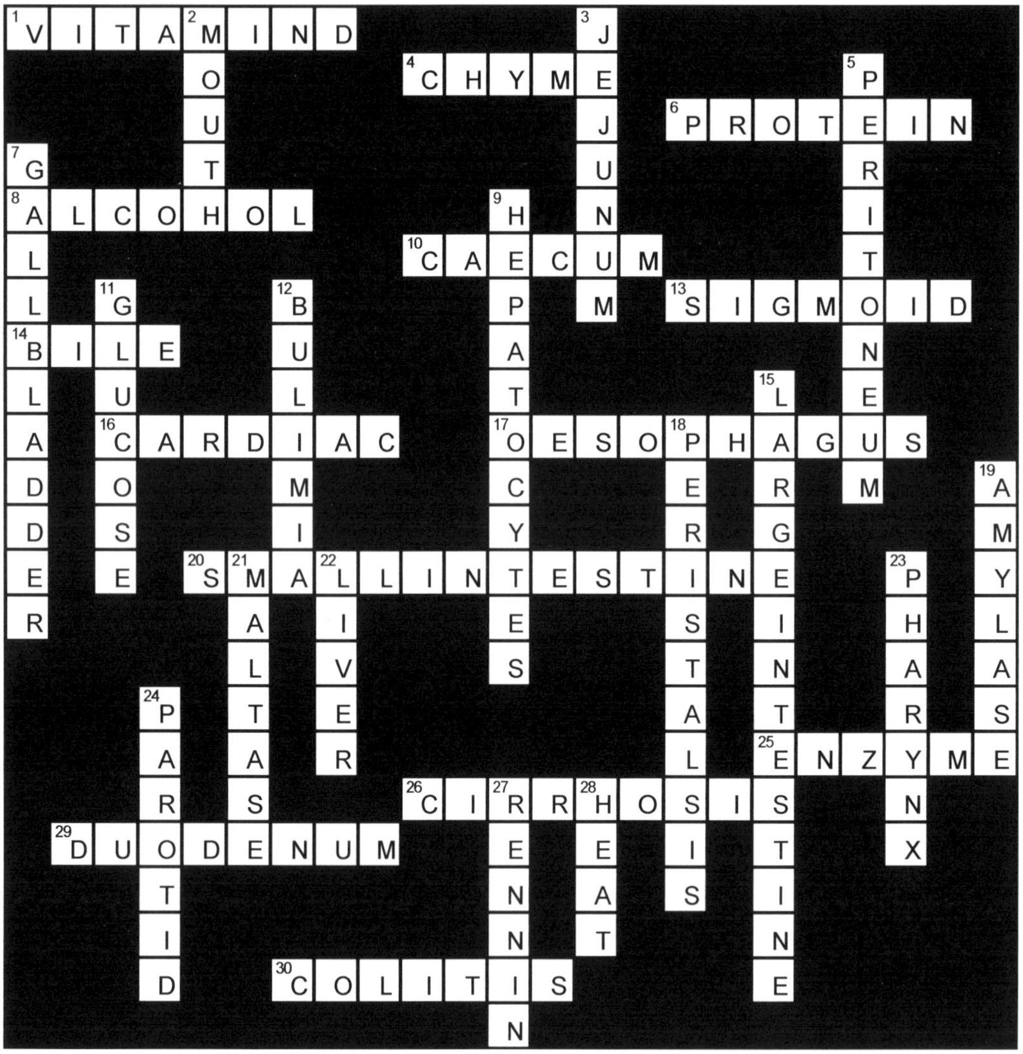
1 VITAMIND
2 MOUTH
3 JEJUNUM
4 CHYME
5 PERITONEUM
6 PROTEIN
7 GALLBLADDER
8 ALCOHOL
9 HEPATOCYTES
10 CAECUM
11 GLUCOSE
12 BULIMIA
13 SIGMOID
14 BILE
15 LARGEINTESTINE
16 CARDIAC
17 OESOPHAGUS
18 PERISTALSIS
19 AMYLASE
20 SMALLINTESTINE
21 MALTASE
22 LIVER
23 PHARYNX
24 PAROTID
25 ENZYME
26 CIRRHOSIS
27 RENNIN
28 HEAT
29 DUODENUM
30 COLITIS

Exercise 4 (fill in the missing words):

1. Stomach
2. Bile
3. Accessory
4. Large
5. Pyloric
6. Submandibular
7. Protein
8. Mucus
9. Fats
10. Carbohydrate
11. Water
12. Epiglottis
13. Villi
14. Ileum
15. Emulsifies
16. Small
17. Papillae
18. Mouth
19. Energy
20. Amylase

Exercise 5 (word search):

1. Mechanical
2. Amino Acids
3. Rectum
4. External
5. Pancreas
6. Enzymes
7. Colon
8. Bile
9. Lipase
10. Lactase
11. Lacteal
12. Liver
13. Hydrochloric Acid
14. Stomach
15. Sublingual
16. Alcohol
17. Duodenum
18. Intestinal Juice
19. Peptidases
20. Ileum

Exercise 6 (match the digestive enzymes with their corresponding functions):

1. Pepsin
2. Peptidases
3. Hydrochloric Acid
4. Sucrase
5. Glucose
6. Salivary Amylase
7. Fatty Acids & Glycerol
8. Trypsin
9. Maltase
10. Lipase

Exercise 7 (multiple choice questions):

1	A	9	B	17	B	25	B	33	A
2	C	10	A	18	D	26	D	34	B
3	D	11	A	19	A	27	C	35	C
4	C	12	D	20	C	28	D	36	A
5	A	13	B	21	A	29	C	37	A
6	C	14	D	22	B	30	A	38	C
7	B	15	D	23	A	31	C	39	B
8	D	16	B	24	B	32	D	40	B

Chapter 12 | The Urinary System

Revision Puzzles & Questions

Exercise 1

The following grid lists statements on the left that are either true or false. Please choose your answer on the right. All answers are provided at the end of the chapter.

1.	The ureters transport urine from the urethra to the kidneys	True ☐ False ☐
2.	Lymphoid tissue makes up a layer of the bladder	True ☐ False ☐
3.	The kidneys are positioned on the posterior wall of the abdomen	True ☐ False ☐
4.	The composition of urine is 98% water, 1% urea and 1% other substances	True ☐ False ☐
5.	Inflammation of the kidney is known as nephritis	True ☐ False ☐
6.	The loop of henle arises from the distal convoluted tubules	True ☐ False ☐
7.	The renal pelvis collects urine from the renal pyramids in the medulla	True ☐ False ☐

Anatomy & Physiology Student Workbook

8.	The urethra passes from the bladder to the outside of the body	True ☐ False ☐
9.	Nephrons are found in the bladder	True ☐ False ☐
10.	The urinary bladder stores urine	True ☐ False ☐
11.	Blood and lymphatic vessels enter the kidneys via the helium	True ☐ False ☐
12.	The ureters consist of an outer layer of muscular tissue	True ☐ False ☐
13.	The glomerulus filters the waste	True ☐ False ☐
14.	The process of expelling urine from the bladder is known as micturition	True ☐ False ☐
15.	The kidneys connect the medulla to the ureter	True ☐ False ☐
16.	Inflammation of the bladder is known as cystitis	True ☐ False ☐
17.	The Bowman's Capsule surrounds the convoluted tubules	True ☐ False ☐

18.	The kidneys are made up of an inner part called the cortex	True ☐ False ☐
19.	Urine is propelled from the kidneys into the bladder by peristalsis	True ☐ False ☐
20.	Blood enters the medulla of the kidney from the efferent arterioles	True ☐ False ☐

Exercise 2

Complete the following crossword on The Urinary System by answering the clues below.

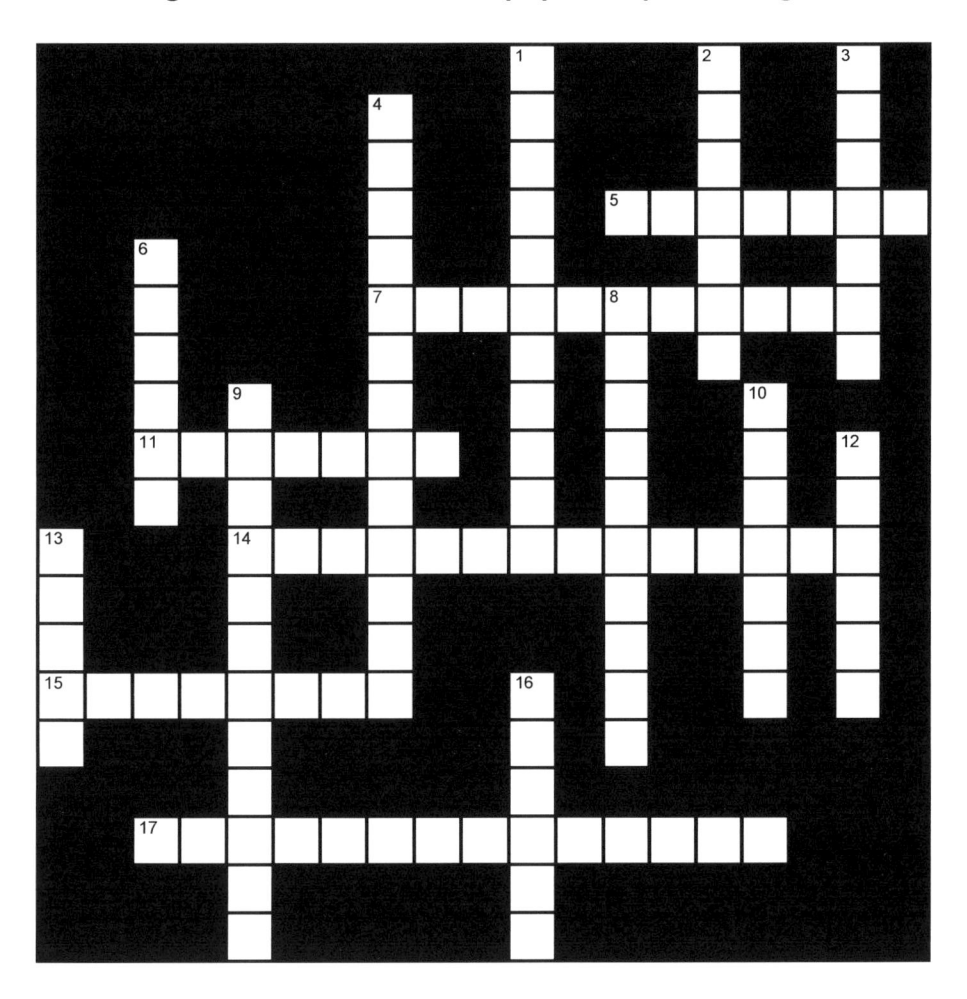

Across
5. What is responsible for controlling the amount of water found within the blood? (7)
7. What do the proximal convoluted tubules straighten out to form? (11)
11. What passes the urine from the bladder to outside the body? (7)
14. What surrounds the glomerulus? (14)
15. Tiny twisted tubes that carry out the filtration and excretion work of the kidneys (8)
17. Inflammation of the kidneys (14)

Down
1. Collects urine from the renal pyramids in the medulla and passes it into the ureters (11)
2. A pear shaped organ found in the pelvic cavity (7)
3. What part of the renal pelvis connects with the top of the pyramids of the medulla? (7)
4. What structures are found inside the medulla of the kidneys? (13)
6. What type of membrane forms an inner lining around the bladder? (6)
8. A process by which urine is processed (10)

9. A function of the kidneys (12)
10. What is the inner section of the kidneys called? (7)
12. A muscular tube that carries urine from the renal pelvis to the bladder (6)
13. A liquid produced by the urinary system after filtration and re-absorption takes place (5)
16. Through what part of the kidney does the ureter enter? (6)

Exercise 3

The flow of urine travels through a series of stages before it is excreted from the body. Please match the stages in the table below. Stage 1 has been completed for you.

1.	Nephron	Stage 1
2.	Urethra	
3.	Ureter	
4.	Outside the body	
5.	Renal Pelvis	
6.	Bladder	

Exercise 4

Fill in the missing words

1. Blood that needs to be processed enters the _____ of the kidney (7)

2. The ureter carries urine from the _____ to the bladder (7)

3. The urinary system is made up of the kidneys, ureters, _____ and the urethra (7)

4. The _____ system works closely with the urinary system to ensure the correct filtration of blood (11)

5. The urethra has an external sphincter which is under _____ control (9)

6. The urinary system is responsible for removing waste products such as alcohol and _____ (4)

7. The renal pelvis collects urine from the _____ _____ in the medulla and passes it into the ureter (5,8)

8. The tubules of the nephron that lead away from the Bowman's Capsule are called _____ convoluted tubules (8)

9. The kidneys are responsible for _____ the blood (9)

10. The excretion of urine from the body is known as _____ (11)

11. Nephritis is _____ of the kidneys (12)

12. Substances that are needed by the body that are found with the waste, such as vitamins, amino acids and glucose are _____ into the bloodstream (10)

13. The bladder is responsible for _____ urine (7)

14. The upper surface of the bladder is composed of a layer of _____ membrane (6)

15. Re-absorption takes place in the _____ (7)

Exercise 5

Please answer the questions below and find the answers in the word search puzzle.

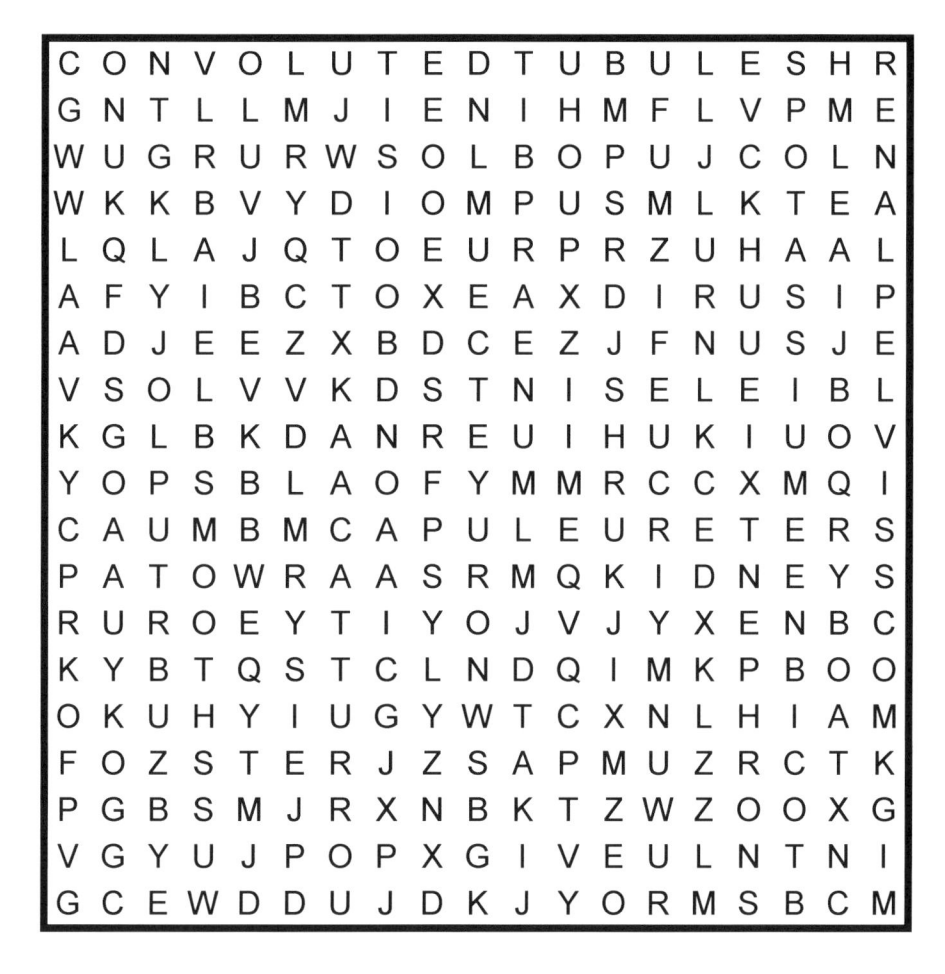

```
C O N V O L U T E D T U B U L E S H R
G N T L L M J I E N I H M F L V P M E
W U G R U R W S O L B O P U J C O L N
W K K B V Y D I O M P U S M L K T E A
L Q L A J Q T O E U R P R Z U H A A L
A F Y I B C T O X E A X D I R U S I P
A D J E E Z X B D C E Z J F N U S J E
V S O L V V K D S T N I S E L E I B L
K G L B K D A N R E U I H U K I U O V
Y O P S B L A O F Y M M R C C X M Q I
C A U M B M C A P U L E U R E T E R S
P A T O W R A A S R M Q K I D N E Y S
R U R O E Y T I Y O J V J Y X E N B C
K Y B T Q S T C L N D Q I M K P B O O
O K U H Y I U G Y W T C X N L H I A M
F O Z S T E R J Z S A P M U Z R C T K
P G B S M J R X N B K T Z W Z O O X G
V G Y U J P O P X G I V E U L N T N I
G C E W D D U J D K J Y O R M S B C M
```

1. What part of the kidney filters fluid from the blood? (11)
2. What is formed in the kidneys? (5)
3. What collects the waste products that are carried in the blood? (14)
4. What disorder of the urinary system causes pain when urinating? (8)
5. A substance found in urine (9)
6. What part of the urinary system stores urine? (7)
7. Blood filtration tubes (8)
8. What organs receive unfiltered blood from the body? (7)
9. A network of tiny blood vessels inside the nephron (10)
10. What receives the filtered substances from the Bowman's Capsule? (17)
11. What receives the urine before it is emptied into the ureter? (11)
12. What muscular tubes connect the kidneys to the bladder? (7)
13. A stage of urine production (10)
14. What type of muscle tissue is found in the ureters? (6)
15. What is urine mainly composed of? (5)

Exercise 6

The process of filtration, re-absorption and collection goes through 8 main stages. Please match the stages in the table below. Stage 1 has been completed for you.

1.	Medulla	Stage 1
2.	Proximal Convoluted Tubules	
3.	Distal Convoluted Tubes	
4.	Bowman's Capsule	
5.	Loop of Henle	
6.	Glomerulus	
7.	Renal Pelvis	
8.	Ureter	

Exercise 7

Multiple choice questions, please choose one answer from the 4 choices in each box.

1. Which one of the following is not a function of the kidneys? a) Re-absorption of substances needed by the body b) To filter blood c) To form urine d) To store urine Answer	2. What part of the urinary system extends from the bladder to outside the body? a) Urethra b) Renal pelvis c) Ureter d) Medulla Answer
3. What are the blood filtration units found inside the kidneys? a) Glomerulus b) Tubules c) Pyramids d) Nephrons Answer	4. Which one of the following systems is not part of the excretory system? a) Skin b) Digestive c) Skeletal d) Respiratory Answer
5. What surrounds the glomerulus? a) Renal pelvis b) Bowman's capsule c) Nephrons d) Distal convoluted tubules Answer	6. What is the composition of urine? a) 98% water, 1% urea, 1% other substances b) 95% water, 2% urea, 3% other substances c) 94% water, 3% urea, 3% other substances d) 96% water, 2% urea, 2% other substances Answer
7. Why is cystitis more common in females? a) Women have shorter ureters b) Women have a shorter urethra c) Women produce more ADH d) Women have smaller bladders Answer	8. Which one of the following is not a process of urine production? a) Filtration b) Collection c) Excretion d) Re-absorption Answer

9. On average, how many litres of urine is produced every day?
a) 1 litre
b) 3 litres
c) 1-2 litres
d) 0.5 litres

Answer
_____

10. What extends from the proximal convoluted tubules?
a) Loop of henle
b) Bowman's Capsule
c) Distal convoluted tubules
d) Renal pelvis

Answer
_____

11. Where are the kidneys positioned?
a) Anterior wall of the abdomen
b) Posterior wall of the abdomen
c) Posterior wall of the pelvic cavity
d) Above the stomach on either side of the spine

Answer
_____

12. What part of the urinary system stores urine?
a) Bladder
b) Ureters
c) Urethra
d) Kidneys

Answer
_____

13. What is the outside part of the kidney called?
a) Hilium
b) Medulla
c) Pelvis
d) Cortex

Answer
_____

14. What gives urine its colour?
a) Oxygen
b) Biliruben
c) Haemoglobin
d) Salt

Answer
_____

15. What are the tubes that lead away from the Bowman's capsule from the nephrons?
a) Proximal convoluted tubules
b) Pelvic calyces
c) Distal convoluted tubules
d) Renal pyramids

Answer
_____

16. Which one of the following is a layer of tissue of the ureters?
a) Skeletal muscle tissue
b) Smooth muscle tissue
c) Adipose tissue
d) Yellow elastic tissue

Answer
_____

17. What hormone is responsible for the amount of water reabsorbed within the blood? a) ADH b) HGH c) ACTH d) MSH Answer _____	18. What connects the medulla to the ureter? a) Kidneys b) Bladder c) Renal pelvis d) Renal pyramids Answer _____
19. Inflammation of the kidneys is known as; a) Cystitis b) Phlebitis c) Nephritis d) Rhinitis Answer _____	20. Why are substances forced through the walls of the glomerulus? a) Because the pressure is high b) Because the blood content is high c) Because there are large levels of waste products d) Because there are high levels of carbon dioxide Answer _____

The Urinary System

Answers

Exercise 1 (true/false):

1. False	11. True
2. False	12. False
3. True	13. True
4. False	14. True
5. True	15. False
6. False	16. True
7. True	17. False
8. True	18. False
9. False	19. True
10. True	20. False

Exercise 2 (crossword):

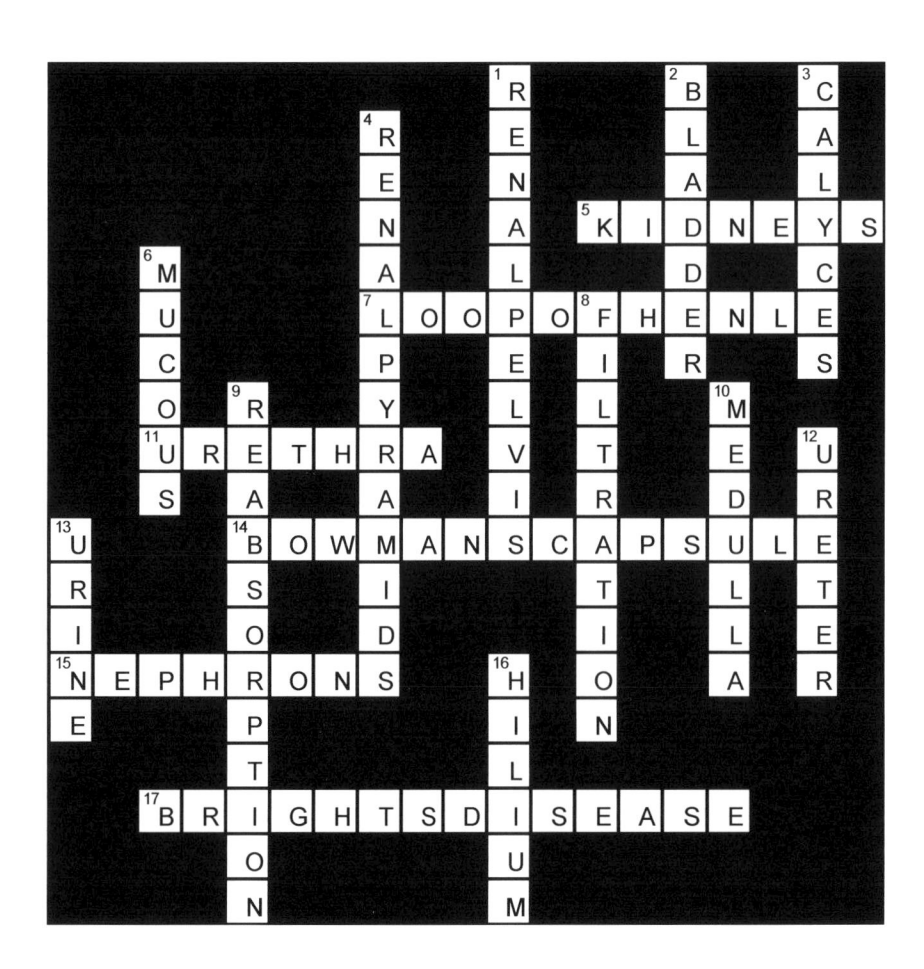

Across:
- 5. KIDNEYS
- 7. LOOPOFHENLE
- 11. URETHRA
- 14. BOWMANSCAPSULE
- 15. NEPHRONS
- 17. BRIGHTSDISEASE

Down:
- 1. RENAL
- 2. BLADDER
- 3. CALYCES
- 4. RENALPELVIS
- 6. MUCOSA
- 8. FILTRATE
- 9. RAA (RENIN)
- 10. MEDULLA
- 12. URETER
- 13. URINE
- 14. BSOIDPT
- 16. HILUM

Exercise 3 (match the stages of the flow of urine until it is excreted from the body):
1. Stage 1
2. Stage 5
3. Stage 3
4. Stage 6
5. Stage 2
6. Stage 4

Exercise 4 (fill in the missing words):
1. Medulla
2. Kidneys
3. Bladder
4. Circulatory
5. Voluntary
6. Urea
7. Renal Pyramids
8. Proximal
9. Filtering
10. Micturition
11. Inflammation
12. Reabsorbed
13. Storing
14. Serous
15. Tubules

Exercise 5 (word search):
1. Outer Cortex
2. Urine
3. Bowman's Capsule
4. Cystitis
5. Potassium
6. Bladder
7. Nephrons
8. Kidneys
9. Glomerulus
10. Convoluted Tubules
11. Renal Pelvis
12. Ureters
13. Collection
14. Smooth
15. Water

Exercise 6 (match the process of urine filtration, re-absorption and collection with each stage it goes through):
1. Stage 1
2. Stage 4
3. Stage 6
4. Stage 3
5. Stage 5
6. Stage 2
7. Stage 7
8. Stage 8

Exercise 7 (multiple choice questions):

1	D	9	C	17	A
2	A	10	A	18	C
3	D	11	B	19	C
4	C	12	A	20	A
5	B	13	D		
6	D	14	B		
7	B	15	A		
8	C	16	B		

Anatomy & Physiology Student Workbook

Chapter 13 | Mock Exam Papers

Paper 1

01. What is the function of endoplasmic reticulum?		Answer
a) To transport substances from one part of a cell to another	b) Growth & repair	
c) Destroys worn out parts of a cell	d) Secretes carbohydrates	
02. Which type of cartilage is found on the surfaces of joints?		Answer
a) Hyaline	b) Yellow elastic	
c) Elastic	d) White fibrocartilage	
03. What do Mast Cells produce?		Answer
a) Areolar tissue	b) Histamine & heparin	
c) Melanin	d) Red blood cells	
04. In which layer of the epidermis does mitosis occur?		Answer
a) Prickle cell layer	b) Granular layer	
c) Basal layer	d) Clear layer	
05. Which of the following skin disorders is contagious?		Answer
a) Impetigo	b) Acne vulgaris	
c) Chloasma	d) Comedones	
06. What bones form the bridge of the nose?		Answer
a) Ethmoid bones	b) Nasal bones	
c) Vomer	d) Lacrimal	
07. Inflammation of the joints is known as;		Answer
a) Gout	b) Osteoporosis	
c) Neuritis	d) Arthritis	
08. What cells break down areas of bone tissue?		Answer
a) Osteoblasts	b) Osteocytes	
c) Osteoclasts	d) Chondrocytes	
09. Which of the following is not an action of the pectoralis major?		Answer
a) Draws arm backwards	b) Draws arm forwards	
c) Medially rotates arm	d) Adducts humerus	

10. What is the composition of muscle?		Answer
a) 75% water, 20% protein, 5% mineral salts, fats and glycogen	b) 75% water, 15% protein, 10% mineral salts, fats and glucose	
c) 75% water, 20% protein, 5% mineral salts, fats and maltase	d) 75% water and 25% protein	
11. What muscle elevates the mandible?		Answer
a) Sternocleidomastoid	b) Medial pterygoid	
c) Lateral pterygoid	d) Buccinator	
12. Which one of the following is not a function of superficial fascia?		Answer
a) Helps retain body warmth	b) Connects skin with deep fascia	
c) Allows movement of the skin	d) Connects muscles with deep fascia	
13. The function of monocytes is to;		Answer
a) Destroy harmful blood cells to protect the body from infection	b) Transport oxygen as oxyhaemoglobin around the body	
c) Defend the system against micro-organisms	d) Eat bacteria and other micro-organisms	
14. Pulmonary circulation is the transport of blood;		Answer
a) From the lungs to the heart	b) From the heart to the upper and lower body	
c) From the heart to the lungs	d) From the lungs to the heart and back again	
15. What is tachycardia?		Answer
a) A heart pain caused by lack of oxygen to the heart	b) A blockage in the pulmonary artery	
c) A blood clot in the coronary artery	d) A particularly rapid heartbeat	
16. An efferent lymphatic vessel transports lymph;		Answer
a) To the lymphatic ducts	b) Back to the system	
c) To the lymph nodes	d) To the lymphatic vessels	
17. What is the function of glucocorticoids?		Answer
a) Regulates thyroid gland	b) Controls male sex hormones	
c) Metabolises proteins, carbohydrates and fats	d) Regulates basic metabolic rate	
18. Which hormone is produced by the pineal gland?		Answer
a) Glucogen	b) Melatonin	
c) Adrenaline	d) Parathormone	

19. Hyposecretion of insulin and glucagon causes;		Answer
a) Hypoglycaemia	b) Diabetes insipidus	
c) Sweating	d) Diabetes mellitus	
20. How many pairs of cranial nerves are there?		Answer
a) 8	b) 12	
c) 5	d) 31	
21. The brain stem is made up of 3 parts;		Answer
a) Hypothalamus, midbrain, medulla oblongata	b) Midbrain, pons varolii, medulla oblongata	
c) Hypothalamus, pons varolii, medulla oblongata	d) Midbrain, pons varolii, hypothalamus	
22. The gap where one neuron meets another neuron is called;		Answer
a) Synapse	b) Neurilemma	
c) Axon	d) Nodes of ranvier	
23. Where does the epididymis begin?		Answer
a) Below the scrotum	b) At the end of the prostate gland	
c) At the top rear of each testis	d) Between the urethra and bladder	
24. Where does fertilization take place in the female reproductive system?		Answer
a) Uterus	b) Fallopian tubes	
c) Urethra	d) Ovaries	
25. What is the function of bile?		Answer
a) The breakdown of proteins	b) The breakdown of glycerol	
c) The breakdown of bacteria	d) To break down fats	
26. What is the function of the small intestine?		Answer
a) To absorb nutrients into the bloodstream	b) To emulsify fats and carbohydrates	
a) To remove waste	d) To begin the production of intestinal juices	
27. What is the structure of bronchi?		Answer
a) Hyaline cartilage and smooth muscle	b) Hyaline cartilage and voluntary muscle	
c) Hyaline cartilage and elastic tissue	d) Hyaline cartilage and cardiac muscle	
28. What is the inner layer of the pleura called?		Answer
a) Parietal layer	b) Palatine layer	
c) Visceral layer	d) Serous layer	

29. Parturition is another term for;		Answer
a) Expiration	b) Giving birth	
c) Discharge of faeces	d) Discharge of urine	
30. Where does each kidney excrete urine?		Answer
a) Renal pelvis	b) Bladder	
c) Urethra	d) Ureter	
31. A group of tissues join to form;		Answer
a) Organ	b) System	
c) Organism	d) Cells	
32. At the anaphase of mitosis the;		Answer
a) The centrioles separate and form spindle fibres	b) Identical pairs of chromosomes move to one end of the cell and the other pairs move to the opposite end of the cell	
c) Centrosome divides into 2 centrioles	d) Cell is resting	
33. Which one of the following is the protective outer layer of the hair?		Answer
a) Outer root sheath	b) Medulla	
c) Cuticle	d) Cortex	
34. Onychophagy describes;		Answer
a) Egg shell nails	b) Hang nails	
c) Ringworm	d) Bitten nails	
35. Define synovitis;		Answer
a) A congenital disorder of the vertebral column	b) Inflammation of a synovial membrane that lines a joint	
c) An auto immune disease that attacks the synovial joints	d) A type of arthritis which causes the spine to become rigid	
36. What is the structure of muscle tissue?		Answer
a) Muscle tissue has spindle shaped cells with a nucleus	b) Muscle tissue is bound together in bundles and enclosed in a sheath	
c) Muscle tissue has striated fibres with only 1 nucleus	d) Muscle tissue is made up of several nuclei and is enclosed by a sheath	
37. Where is the coracobrachialis positioned?		Answer
a) Lower arm	b) Elbow	
c) Humerus	d) Anterior forearm	

38. Lack of tone in a muscle is known as;		Answer
a) Myositis	b) Atony	
c) Atrophy	d) Rupture	
39. Which one of the following is one of the main arteries of the head and neck?		Answer
a) Right renal artery	b) Hepatic artery	
c) Maxillary	d) External carotid	
40. What protein gives blood its red colour?		Answer
a) Fibrinogen	b) Haemoglobin	
c) Albumin	d) Platelets	
41. Lymphatic vessels open up into;		Answer
a) Lymph nodes	b) Lymph duct	
c) Lymph tissue	d) Lymph capillaries	
42. What is the function of calcitonin?		Answer
a) Helps glucose enter cells	b) Controls body rhythms	
c) Controls calcium levels in the blood	d) Sexual development	
43. Which one of the following is a function of the sympathetic nervous system?		Answer
a) Constricts blood flow to the heart	b) Causes dilation of skeletal blood vessels	
c) Slows down the heart rate	d) Releases acetylcholine	
44. A loss of dopamine occurs when an individual is suffering from;		Answer
a) Multiple sclerosis	b) Parkinson's disease	
c) Cerebral palsy	d) Myalgic encephalomyelitis	
45. What are the male gonads called?		Answer
a) Prostate gland	b) Epididymis	
c) Testes	d) Testicular vessels	
46. Where is the gall bladder positioned?		Answer
a) Behind the liver	b) In front of the liver	
c) To the left of the liver	d) To the right of the liver	
47. Which one of the following is not stored by the liver?		Answer
a) Iron	b) Vitamin E	
c) Glycogen	d) Vitamin B6	
48. What forms the Adam's Apple?		Answer
a) Small masses of lymphoid tissue	b) The thyroid cartilage surrounding the larynx	
c) Pharyngeal tonsils	d) Palatine tonsils	

49. What is the function of the Bowman's Capsule?		Answer
a) Absorption of waste products	b) Acts as a passageway for urine through the kidneys	
c) Acts as the first step for filtering blood in the kidneys	d) To carry waste products from the glomerulus to the loop of henle	
50. What is the structure of the bladder?		Answer
a) A funnel shaped organ	b) A funnel shaped cavity	
c) A bean shaped organ	d) A hollow sac like organ	

Paper 2

1. What does cytoplasm not contain?		Answer
a) Mitochondria	b) Ribosomes	
c) Nucleus	d) Endoplasmic reticulum	
2. The spindle fibres disappear during which phase of mitosis?		Answer
a) Metaphase	b) Prophase	
c) Interphase	d) Telophase	
3. What is the function of the nucleolus?		Answer
a) The control the centre of the cell	b) To produce chromosomes	
c) To produce protein	d) Form ribosomes	
4. Erector pili can be defined as;		Answer
a) Hair follicles which produce sebum	b) Small muscles which are attached to each hair follicle	
c) Microscopic capillaries	d) Nerve endings	
5. Where is terminal hair found?		Answer
a) On a foetus	b) Eyebrows	
c) Eyelids	d) Soles of the feet	
6. The Acid Mantle is formed from;		Answer
a) Eccrine & apocrine fluid	b) Mast cells	
c) Sweat & sebum	d) Histamine & heparin	
7. What is dermatitis?		Answer
a) An inflammation of the skin caused by contact with external factors	b) An allergy marked by the eruption of wheals with severe itching	
c) An erythema covered with silvery scales	d) Eczema	
8. The perionychium describes;		Answer
a) The extension of the nail plate beyond the nail bed	b) The skin that adheres to the base of the nail	
c) The cuticles that overlap the sides of the nail	d) The deep fold of skin at the base of the nail	
9. Which bone joins the foot to the leg?		Answer
a) Navicular	b) Cuboid	
c) Cuneiform	d) Talus	
10. The fibula is a type of;		Answer
a) Short bone	b) Irregular bone	
c) Flat bone	d) Long bone	

Anatomy & Physiology Student Workbook

11. What parts of the body does the axial skeleton support?		Answer
a) Head and neck	b) Lower limbs	
c) Head, neck, spine, ribs and sternum	d) Shoulder girdle and upper limbs	
12. Which bone divides the nose into the left and right halves?		Answer
a) Vomer	b) Sphenoid	
c) Parietal	d) Lacrimal	
13. The anatomical term, palmar, refers to;		Answer
a) The palm of the hand	b) The inner surface of the body	
c) The sole of the foot	d) Lying face up	
14. Which muscle helps to bend the neck laterally?		Answer
a) Mentalis	b) Ilio psoas	
c) Levator scapulae	d) Masseter	
15. Which muscle flexes the wrist?		Answer
a) Flexor carpi digitorum	b) Flexor digitorum superficialis	
c) Brachioradialis	d) Flexor carpi radialis	
16. Which of the following is an involuntary action?		Answer
a) Lifting an arm	b) Heartbeat	
c) Medially rotates humerus	d) Moving fingers	
17. What is the structure of voluntary muscle?		Answer
a) Bundles of nerve cells surrounded by unmyelinated sheath	b) Spindle shaped cells with no nucleus	
c) Bundles of muscle fibres surrounded by a sheath	d) Striated fibres with a membrane and nucleus	
18. Which one of the following is not an action of the teres major?		Answer
a) Rotates scapula	b) Adducts humerus	
c) Medially rotates humerus	d) Extends shoulder joint	
19. The four plasma proteins are as follows;		Answer
a) Albumin, globulin, fibrinogen and prothrombin	b) Potassium, globulin, albumin and prothrombin	
c) Albumin, potassium, fibrinogen and prothrombin	d) Iodine, prothrombin, fibrinogen and albumin	
20. A haemorrhage occurs when;		Answer
a) A capillary bleeds	b) No blood clot forms	
c) A blood clot is formed	d) There is high blood pressure	

Anatomy & Physiology Student Workbook

21. Pulmonary circulation is the transport of blood;		Answer
a) From the lungs to the heart	b) From the heart to the upper and lower body	
c) From the heart to the lungs	b) From the heart to the upper and lower body	
22. What is the wall that separates the right and left sides of the heart called?		Answer
a) Pericardium	b) Endocardium	
c) Myocardium	d) Septum	
23. What is the function of the right lymphatic duct?		Answer
a) Drains lymph into the head, neck and torso	b) Collects lymph from the right side of the body	
c) Collects lymph from the right side of the head and neck, chest and right arm	d) Collects lymph from the left side of the body	
24. The inguinal nodes are located;		Answer
a) Groin area	b) Behind the knees	
c) Elbows	d) Armpits	
25. What is the function of insulin and glucagon?		Answer
a) Regulates salts in the body	b) Maintains calcium levels in the body	
c) Stabilise blood sugar levels	d) Regulates water absorption	
26. Hyposecretion of thyroxine causes;		Answer
a) Cretinism	b) Amenorrhoea	
c) Sweating	d) Fatigue	
27. Hypersecretion of ADH causes;		Answer
a) Oedema	b) Grave's disease	
c) Diabetes insipidus	d) Cretinism	
28. Which of the following is not one of the main sections of the brain?		Answer
a) The cervical plexus	b) The brain stem	
c) The cerebrum	d) The cerebellum	
29. Which system of the body helps the nervous system to maintain homeostasis?		Answer
a) Respiratory system	b) Endocrine system	
c) Muscular system	d) Circulatory system	
30. Efferent nerves only transmit to which type of tissue?		Answer
a) Muscular tissue	b) Elastic tissue	
c) Muscular and glandular tissue	d) Connective tissue	

31. Where are the testes positioned?		Answer
a) Between the bladder and epididymis	b) At the top of the urethra	
c) At the start of the ureter	d) Within the scrotum	
32. Extremely painful menstruation is known as;		Answer
a) Amenorrhoea	b) Pre menstrual syndrome	
c) Dysmenorrhoea	d) Polycystic ovarian syndrome	
33. The vulva can be defined as;		Answer
a) The external genitalia of the female reproductive system	b) The internal genitalia of the female reproductive system	
c) Mature follicles	d) Female sex cells	
34. What organ secretes intestinal juices?		Answer
a) Small intestine	b) Liver	
c) Gall bladder	d) Pancreas	
35. The stomach is responsible for which type of digestion?		Answer
a) Protein digestion	b) Fat digestion	
c) Carbohydrate digestion	d) Fat and carbohydrate digestion	
36. What leads to the respiratory bronchioles?		Answer
a) Fibrous bronchioles	b) End bronchioles	
c) Terminal bronchioles	d) Ciliated bronchioles	
37. The pharynx opens into the;		Answer
a) Trachea and larynx	b) Oesophagus and trachea	
c) Oesophagus and larynx	d) Trachea and bronchi	
38. What are the 2 layers of the pleura separated by?		Answer
a) Pleura	b) Pleura membrane	
c) Pleura septum	d) Pleural cavity	
39. The muscular tubes which connect the kidneys to the bladder are;		Answer
a) Ureters	b) Urethra	
c) Renal pelvis	d) Hilium	
40. Which one of the following is not a function of the kidney?		Answer
a) Urine production	b) Reabsorption of substances such as glucose and amino acids	
c) Filtration of blood	d) Absorption of water	
41. The turbinator bone is located on which part of the face?		Answer
a) Cheek	b) Nose	
c) Chin	d) Forehead	

42. A compound fracture describes;		Answer
a) The broken part of the bone protruding through the skin	b) A partial fracture of a bone occurring in children only	
c) The broken bone penetrates tissue or organs around it	d) A broken bone in 2 or more places	
43. What is the action of the sternocleidomastoid?		Answer
a) Elevates scapula	b) Draws scapula backwards	
c) Bends neck laterally	d) Flexes head	
44. What is the composition of muscle?		Answer
a) 75% water, 20% protein, 5% mineral salts, fats and glycogen	b) 75% water, 15% protein, 10% mineral salts, fats and glucose	
c) 75% water, 20% protein, 5% mineral salts, fats and maltase	d) 75% water and 25% protein	
45. Where is ATP produced?		Answer
a) Nucleus	b) Nucleolus	
c) Mitochondria	d) Ribosomes	
46. The action of the heart is controlled by;		Answer
a) The central nervous system	b) The autonomic nervous system	
c) The spinal cord	d) The peripheral nervous system	
47. What is the structure of arteries?		Answer
a) They have thick muscular walls and a small lumen	b) They have thin muscular walls and a small lumen	
c) They have thin muscular walls and a thin lumen	d) They have thin elastic walls and a large lumen	
48. A simple sugar is known as;		Answer
a) Monosaccharide	b) Polysaccharide	
c) Saccharide	d) Disaccharide	
49. The alveoli arise from;		Answer
a) Bronchioles	b) Bronchi	
c) Pleural cavity	d) Larynx	
50. What is the function of bronchi?		Answer
a) To exchange gases	b) To carry air from the trachea into the bronchioles	
c) To begin inhalation	d) To filter bacteria	

Paper 3

1. What is a cell mainly composed of?		Answer
a) Cytoplasm	b) Centrioles	
c) Water	d) Mitochondria	
2. What is the function of hyaline cartilage?		Answer
a) Helps to maintain the shape of an area	b) Flexibility & support	
c) To add nutrients to articulating surfaces	d) Stretch & recoil	
3. The study of the structure of the body is known as;		Answer
a) Histology	b) Homeostasis	
c) Physiology	d) Anatomy	
4. Osmosis describes;		Answer
a) The process of moving small molecules such as oxygen and carbon dioxide through the cell membrane	b) The process of moving water through the cell membrane from an area of high concentration to an area of low concentration or vice versa	
c) The movement of water across a membrane	d) The transfer of glucose and amino acids through the cell membrane to equal concentration	
5. Desquamation can be defined as;		Answer
a) The dead skin cells on the surface of the skin are constantly shedding	b) Granules which are visible in healing after trauma	
c) A pigmentation which gives skin its colour	d) Cell division	
6. Which skin disorder affects the forehead, cheeks and nose, causing a flushed reddened appearance?		Answer
a) Acne vulgaris	b) Eczema	
c) Herpes zoster	d) Acne rosacea	
7. The stratum lucidum is known as;		Answer
a) Clear layer	b) Surface layer	
c) Basal layer	d) Granular layer	
8. Which pigment gives skin its natural colour?		Answer
a) Histamine	b) Melanin	
c) Heparin	d) Collagen	
9. What part of the hair lies above the skin's surface?		Answer
a) Root	b) Bulb	
c) Shaft	d) Matrix	

10. Which of the following can be found in the epidermis?		Answer
a) Sweat glands	b) Lymph vessels	
c) Melanocytes	d) Elastin	
11. Haversian canals can be defined as;		Answer
a) Small channels running lengthways	b) Small channels running lengthways through compact bone	
c) Small channels running lengthways through cancellous bone	d) Small channels found in cancellous bone containing oxygen and nutrients	
12. Where is the foramen magnus located?		Answer
a) Occipital bone	b) Mandible	
c) Parietal bone	d) Frontal	
13. Which part of the body is the cervical spine positioned?		Answer
a) Lower back	b) Ribs	
c) Neck	d) Pelvis	
14. Which type of joint is the least moveable?		Answer
a) Hinge	b) Ball & Socket	
c) Gliding	d) Saddle	
15. How many bones does an adult skeleton have?		Answer
a) 240	b) 206	
c) 160	d) 200	
16. Which muscle raises the eyebrows?		Answer
a) Frontalis	b) Risorius	
c) Procerus nasi	d) Occipitofrontalis	
17. What is the structure of a tendon?		Answer
a) White fibrous elastic tissue	b) White fibrous adipose tissue	
c) White fibrous elastic cords	d) White fibrous inelastic cords	
18. Which one of the following muscles is not part of the quadriceps?		Answer
a) Vastus lateralis	b) Rectus femoris	
c) Biceps femoris	d) Vastus medialis	
19. What muscle elevates the mandible?		Answer
a) Sternocleidomastoid	b) Medial pterygoid	
c) Lateral pterygoid	d) Buccinator	

Anatomy & Physiology Student Workbook

20. When you are looking at a diagram of the heart, the upper left chamber is called the;		Answer
a) Left ventricle	b) Right atria	
c) Right ventricle	d) Left atria	
21. What is the function of leucocytes?		Answer
a) Blood clotting	b) To fight infection	
c) To transport waste products	d) Regulate body temperature	
22. The function of capillaries include;		Answer
a) To deliver oxygen and nutrients to most parts of the body	b) To carry deoxygenated blood from the capillaries to the larger veins	
c) To relax and dilate providing a small blood supply to vital organs	d) To carry oxygenated blood to larger veins	
23. Hepatitis A, B & C affect which organ of the body;		Answer
a) Spleen	b) Pancreas	
c) Heart	d) Liver	
24. Lymphatic capillaries join up to become;		Answer
a) Lymph nodes	b) Lymphatic vessels	
c) Lymphatic tissue	d) Lymphatic ducts	
25. Which one of the following is not a function of the spleen?		Answer
a) Forms new leucocytes	b) Removes foreign particles	
c) Helps fight infection	d) Acts as a blood reservoir	
26. Lymphatic vessels open up into;		Answer
a) Lymph nodes	b) Lymph duct	
c) Lymph tissue	d) Lymph capillaries	
27. Which hormone does the adrenal medulla secrete?		Answer
a) Glucocorticoids	b) Adrenaline	
c) Insulin	d) Testosterone	
28. An endocrine gland;		Answer
a) Is a chemical messenger	b) A ductless gland which produces hormones	
c) A hormone	d) A ductless gland	
29. Hypersecretion of testosterone in women causes;		Answer
a) Cushing's syndrome	b) Amenorrhoea	
c) Addisons disease	d) Breast growth	

30. Where is the pancreas located?		Answer
a) Above the stomach	b) In the abdomen, partially behind the stomach	
c) Behind the lungs	d) In between the lungs	
31. Where are neurilemma found?		Answer
a) Around the axons of peripheral nerves	b) Spinal cord	
c) Brain	d) Autonomic nervous system	
32. A reflex is produced by;		Answer
a) Nerve cells	b) Stimulus	
c) Nerve endings	d) Voluntary movement	
33. What is the function of the spinal cord?		Answer
a) Carries motor nerve fibres to the autonomic nervous system	b) Carries motor and sensory nerve fibres to the peripheral nervous system	
a) Transmits messages to the brain	b) Transmission of nerve signals between the brain and body	
34. Where does the epididymis begin?		Answer
a) Below the scrotum	b) At the end of the prostate gland	
c) At the top rear of each testis	d) Between the urethra and bladder	
35. What is the function of the placenta?		Answer
a) To secrete milk, post pregnancy	b) To allow the passage of nutrients to the baby and waste elimination from the baby	
c) To break down the tail of the sperm after fertilization	d) To enable the foetus to move	
36. How long is the small intestine?		Answer
a) 12.5m	b) 9m	
c) 7m	d) 1.5m	
37. Saliva contains;		Answer
a) Salt, water and bile	b) Water, mucus and enzymes	
c) Water and enzymes	d) Water, mucus and hydrochloric acid	

38. What is the function of the epiglottis?		Answer
a) To digest proteins and carbohydrates	b) To prevent choking	
a) Aids mastication	b) To lubricate the food with water and mucus	
39. What is the structure of bronchi?		Answer
a) Hyaline cartilage and smooth muscle	b) Hyaline cartilage and voluntary muscle	
c) Hyaline cartilage and elastic tissue	d) Hyaline cartilage and cardiac muscle	
40. Which part of the respiratory system is the final passageway of air from the nose to the lungs?		Answer
a) Alveoli	b) Bronchi	
c) Bronchioles	d) Pleura	
41. What is the function of the Bowman's Capsule?		Answer
a) Absorption of waste products	b) Acts as a passageway for urine through the kidneys	
c) Acts as the first step for filtering blood in the kidneys	d) To carry waste products from the glomerulus to the loop of henle	
42. How does blood enter the kidney?		Answer
a) Renal tubule	b) Efferent arteriole	
c) Afferent arteriole	d) Renal artery	
43. What is the renal pelvis?		Answer
a) A bean shaped organ	b) A funnel shaped cavity	
c) A sac like organ	d) A network of vessels	
44. What is the position of the adductor longus?		Answer
a) Front of the thigh	b) Lateral and front of thigh	
c) Lateral front of lower leg	d) Medial side of thigh	
45. The moveable end of a muscle is called;		Answer
a) The insertion	b) The origin	
c) The attachment	d) The belly	
46. What type of fracture occurs when a bone is broken and is driven into another bone?		Answer
a) Greenstick	b) Comminuted	
c) Impacted	d) Simple	
47. Where is bone marrow found?		Answer
a) Compact bone	b) Haversian canals	
c) Cancellous bone	d) Sesamoid bones	

48. What is the PH balance of the skin?		Answer
a) 5.5 - 6.5	b) 5.6 - 6.6	
c) 4.5 - 5.6	d) 5.5 - 6.6	
49. What is the term used to describe ingrown nails?		Answer
a) Onychocryptosis	b) Onychomycosis	
c) Onychophagy	d) Lamella dystrophy	
50. An example of a molecule;		Answer
a) Oxygen	b) Carbon	
c) Hydrogen	d) Carbon Dioxide	

Paper 4

1. Which part of the cell regulates what substances enter and leave a cell?		Answer
a) Cytoplasm	b) Ribosomes	
c) Nucleus	d) Cell membrane	
2. What is the function of the cell membrane?		Answer
a) To control every organelle within the cytoplasm	b) To destroy harmful parts of a cell	
c) To hold the organelles within the cell	d) To let carbohydrates pass through the cell	
3. Phagocytosis describes;		Answer
a) The process used by cells to engulf and destroy harmful bacteria	b) The process used by cells to absorb nutrients and other substances	
c) The process by which cells obtain energy by osmosis	d) The process by which nutrients are released from a cell	
4. Function of yellow elastic cartilage;		Answer
a) Connection	b) Protection	
c) Flexibility	d) Insulation	
5. Inflammation of the tissue surrounding the nails is called;		Answer
a) Onychia	b) Onycholysis	
c) Onychorrhexis	d) Paronychia	
6. Comedones are also known as;		Answer
a) Freckles	b) Hives	
c) Blackheads	d) Whiteheads	
7. What is the purpose of collagen in the skin?		Answer
a) To repair the skin	b) To reduce redness	
c) To produce the anticoagulant heparin	d) To keep the skin firm and elastic	
8. Which one of the following is a layer of the hair?		Answer
a) Cortex	b) Matrix	
c) Dermal papillae	d) Keratin	
9. A non malignant group of pigmented cells;		Answer
a) Mole	b) Naevae	
c) Urticaria	d) Chloasma	
10. Which of the following cells are not found within the dermis?		Answer
a) Leucocytes	b) Mast cells	
c) Thrombocytes	d) Histiocytes	

11. The scapula falls under which category of bone?		Answer
a) Irregular bone	b) Flat bone	
b) Long bone	d) Sesamoid bone	
12. What type of arthritis results in the joints of the spine becoming fused?		Answer
a) Cervical spondylitis	b) Gout	
c) Rheumatoid arthritis	d) Ankylosing spondylitis	
13. How many bones do the lumbar vertebrae contain?		Answer
a) 12	b) 7	
c) 4	d) 5	
14. The anatomical term that describes nearer to the surface is;		Answer
a) Superficial	b) External	
c) Internal	d) Proximal	
15. What are joints?		Answer
a) The location at which 2 or more bones meet	b) The location at which a tendon meets bone	
c) The location at which the origin of a muscle meets its insertion	d) The body's muscles	
16. What is the position of the flexor carpi radialis?		Answer
a) Palm of hand	b) Anterior forearm	
c) Elbow	d) Top of humerus	
17. What muscle lowers the mandible and opens the mouth?		Answer
a) Lateral pterygoid	b) Medial pterygoid	
c) Orbicularis oculi	d) Masseter	
18. What is the strongest muscle in the body?		Answer
a) Deltoids	b) Latissimus dorsi	
c) Hamstrings	d) Gluteus maximus	
19. What is the structure of a tendon?		Answer
a) White fibrous elastic tissue	b) White fibrous adipose tissue	
c) White fibrous elastic cords	d) White fibrous inelastic cords	
20. What is the action of the trapezius?		Answer
a) Flexes head	b) Draws arm forward	
c) Adducts scapula	d) Bend neck laterally	

21. How does the muscular system rely on the respiratory system?		Answer
a) Muscles receive oxygen from the respiratory system for energy	b) Muscles receive glucose from the respiratory system for energy	
c) Muscles receive nerve impulses from the respiratory system for movement	d) Muscles receive glycogen from the respiratory system for heat production	
22. Anaemia can be defined as follows;		Answer
a) A reduction in red blood cells	b) A reduction in white blood cells	
c) An increase in the production of erythrocytes	d) The inability of the blood to clot	
23. Which chamber of the heart does oxygenated blood return to?		Answer
a) Right atrium	b) Left atrium	
c) Right ventricle	d) Left ventricle	
24. What is the main artery that supplies blood to the legs?		Answer
a) Tibial	b) Renal	
c) Brachial	d) Thrombus	
25. A function of arterioles;		Answer
a) To carry oxygenated blood to the lungs	b) To distribute essential waste and bacteria to the body	
c) To carry deoxygenated blood from the capillaries to the larger veins	d) To relax and dilate, speeding up blood flow to the body when needed	
26. Which of the following is not needed for a blood clot to form?		Answer
a) Fibrin	b) Vitamin D	
c) Calcium	d) Prothrombin	
27. What is the relationship between the circulatory and skeletal systems?		Answer
a) Erythrocytes are produced in the red bone marrow of short bones	b) Thrombocytes are produced in the bone marrow of short bones	
c) Erythrocytes are produced in the bone marrow of long bones	d) Erythrocytes are produced in sesamoid bones	
28. Which hormone is produced by the pineal gland?		Answer
a) Glucogen	b) Melatonin	
c) Adrenaline	d) Parathormone	
29. What endocrine gland is located in the centre of the brain?		Answer
a) Pituitary	b) Pineal body	
c) Pancreas	d) Parathyroids	

30. Hyposecretion of HGH causes;		Answer
a) Oedema	b) High blood pressure	
c) Kidney failure	d) Dwarfism	
31. Which part of the brain regulates the actions of the heart and lungs?		Answer
a) Midbrain	b) Hypothalamus	
c) Pons varolii	d) Medulla oblongata	
32. What is the function of neuroglia?		Answer
a) Transmit stimuli to the cell body	b) Supports the neurons	
c) Transmit stimuli away from the cell body	d) Insulates the axon	
33. The bundle of nerves known as the cauda equina are made up of what part of the spinal nerves?		Answer
a) Lumbar, sacral and coccygeal nerves	b) Cervical, thoracic and lumbar nerves	
c) Thoracic, lumbar and sacral nerves	d) Cervical, lumbar and coccygeal nerves	
34. Which one of the following is a function of the cerebrum?		Answer
a) Maintaining homeostasis	b) Controlling conscious movement	
c) Carry messages to the spinal cord	d) Carry messages to and from the brain	
35. What is the first part of the birth canal?		Answer
a) Uterus	b) Cervix	
c) Vagina	d) Fallopian tubes	
36. What is the position of the scrotum?		Answer
a) Above the penis	b) Below the penis	
c) Behind the penis	d) In front of the penis	
37. Which one of the following is not a cause of amenorrhoea?		Answer
a) Congestion of the uterus	b) Hormone imbalances	
c) Extreme weight loss	d) Considerable amounts of exercise	
38. Peptones are broken down into;		Answer
a) Proteins	b) Peptidases	
c) Polypeptides	d) Amino acids	
39. What is the function of bile?		Answer
a) The breakdown of proteins	b) The breakdown of glycerol	
c) The breakdown of bacteria	d) To break down fats	

40. Which one of the following is not a layer of the small intestinal wall?		Answer
a) A layer of blood vessels	b) A layer of fibrous tissue	
c) A muscular layer	d) A layer of lymph vessels	
41. The hollow spaces inside the bones of the skull surrounding the nose are called;		Answer
a) Nasal bones	b) Nasal cavity	
c) Nasal septum	d) Sinuses	
42. Air travels from the pharynx to;		Answer
a) Alveoli	b) Trachea	
c) Bronchi	d) Larynx	
43. The trachea is also known as the;		Answer
a) Voice box	b) Adam's apple	
c) Windpipe	d) Enzyme	
44. Nephritis is a term which describes;		Answer
a) Inflammation of the bladder	b) Inflammation of the gall bladder	
c) Inflammation of the kidney	d) Inflammation of the pelvis	
45. What sphincter controls the flow of urine through the urethra?		Answer
a) Esophageal	b) External	
c) Pyloric	d) Cardiac	
46. Which of the following does not enter the hilium of the kidney?		Answer
a) Urethra	b) Renal vein	
c) Renal artery	d) Renal pelvis	
47. What is the function of the urethra?		Answer
a) To take urine from the bladder to outside the body	b) To store urine	
c) To pass urine from the bladder to the ureter	d) To filter waste	
48. A tear in the fascia surrounding the muscle is called;		Answer
a) Strain	b) Sprain	
c) Rupture	d) Fibrositis	
49. Bending a body part inwards is known as;		Answer
a) Adduction	b) Flexion	
c) Extension	d) Supination	
50. What is the action of the orbicularis oculi?		Answer
a) Opens the eye	b) Closes the eye	
c) Lifts the upper jaw	d) Lifts the lower jaw	

Paper 5

1. What is the energy transporting molecule produced by mitochondria?		Answer
a) ATP	b) Oxygen	
c) Protoplasm	d) Cytoplasm	
2. The study of the structure of the body is known as;		Answer
a) Histology	b) Homeostasis	
c) Physiology	d) Anatomy	
3. What is the process called whereby small molecules, like oxygen and carbon dioxide, can pass through the cell membrane?		Answer
a) Diffusion	b) Osmosis	
c) Filtration	d) Dissolution	
4. What type of skin disorder is impetigo?		Answer
a) Viral infection	b) Congenital infection	
c) Bacterial infection	d) General infection	
5. Ephelides are more commonly referred to as;		Answer
a) Liver spots	b) Whiteheads	
c) Blackheads	d) Freckles	
6. Which one of the following is the middle layer of the hair?		Answer
a) Cortex	b) Shaft	
c) Medulla	d) Bulb	
7. What is the mantle?		Answer
a) The growing area of the nail	b) Deep fold of epidermis just before the cuticle at the base of the nail	
c) The section of skin that the nail plate rests on	d) The grooves at the sides of the nail bed	
8. The bone at the top of the arm is called;		Answer
a) Humerus	b) Ulna	
c) Radius	d) Carpals	
9. What type of joint is the knee?		Answer
a) Gliding	b) Saddle	
c) Hinge	d) Pivot	

10. Which of the following is a type of sesamoid bone?		Answer
a) Maxilla	b) Patella	
c) Humerus	d) Tarsals	
11. What is the shaft of a long bone known as?		Answer
a) Periosteum	b) Diaphysis	
c) Articular cartilage	d) Epiphysis	
12. What parts of the body does the axial skeleton support?		Answer
a) Head and neck	b) Lower limbs	
c) Head, neck , spine, ribs and sternum	d) Shoulder girdle and upper limbs	
13. What muscle is positioned on the front of the lower leg?		Answer
a) Soleus	b) Gastrocnemius	
c) Flexor digitorum longus	d) Tibialis anterior	
14. Which muscle extends the wrist?		Answer
a) Extensor carpi digitorum	b) Pronator teres	
c) Extensor carpi ulnaris	d) Anconeus	
15. What is the action of the vastus medialis?		Answer
a) Flexes knee	b) Extends knee	
c) Flexes hip	d) Extends hip	
16. What is the structure of voluntary muscle?		Answer
a) Bundles of nerve cells surrounded by unmyelinated sheath	b) Spindle shaped cells with no nucleus	
c) Bundles of muscle fibres surrounded by a sheath	d) Striated fibres with a membrane and nucleus	
17. What muscle supports the arches of the feet?		Answer
a) Sartorius	b) Peroneus longus	
c) Tibialis anterior	d) Soleus	
18. Isometric contraction occurs;		Answer
a) When the tension in a muscle increases but its length is not altered	b) When the muscle stretches and moves	
c) When the tension in the muscle remains the same but its length is increased	d) When the muscle contracts	
19. Which muscle is not part of the hamstrings group?		Answer
a) Vastus lateralis	b) Semitendinosus	
c) Biceps femoris	d) Semimembranosus	

20. Anaemia can be defined as follows;		Answer
a) A reduction in red blood cells	b) A reduction in white blood cells	
c) An increase in the production of erythrocytes	d) The inability of the blood to clot	
21. Another term for a heartbeat is;		Answer
a) Systolic pressure	b) Diastolic pressure	
c) Cardiac cycle	d) Pulse	
22. Blood is carried to the lungs via tiny vessels called;		Answer
a) Capillaries	b) Venules	
c) Arteries	d) Arterioles	
23. A sphygmomanometer is used for;		Answer
a) Measuring plasma content	b) Measuring body temperature	
c) Measuring the level of erythrocytes	d) Measuring blood pressure	
24. What is atherosclerosis?		Answer
a) Loss of elasticity in the arterial walls causing a decrease in blood pressure	b) Blood poisoning	
c) Low blood pressure	d) A build up of fats inside the arteries causing them to narrow and harden, limiting blood flow to the body	
25. What is the process by which oxygen can enter the bloodstream?		Answer
a) Absorption	b) Diffusion	
c) Osmosis	d) Filtration	
26. The pulmonary vein carries blood;		Answer
a) From the lungs to the heart	b) From the heart to the rest of the body	
c) From the heart to the lungs	d) From the heart to the upper body	
27. Cancer of the lymphatic tissue is called?		Answer
a) Hodgkin's disease	b) Addison's syndrome	
c) Cushing's syndrome	d) Septicemia	
28. What is the function of lymphatic vessels?		Answer
a) Transport lymph to the spleen	b) Transport lymph to the lymphatic capillaries	
c) Transport lymph to the lymphatic ducts	d) Transport lymph towards the heart	
29. Which one of the following does not help to circulate lymph?		Answer
a) Suction	b) Contraction of skeletal muscles	
c) Heat	d) Pressure	

30. What is the function of glucocorticoids?		Answer
a) Regulates thyroid gland	b) Controls male sex hormones	
c) Metabolises proteins, carbohydrates and fats	d) Regulates basic metabolic rate	
31. The condition in which menstruation stops is known as;		Answer
a) Addison's syndrome	b) Cushing's syndrome	
c) Amenorrhoea	d) Polycystic ovarian syndrome	
32. What hormone regulates the thyroid gland?		Answer
a) Parathormone	b) Thyroid stimulating hormone	
c) Luteinising hormone	d) Insulin	
33. Which hormone does the adrenal medulla secrete?		Answer
a) Glucocorticoids	b) Adrenaline	
c) Insulin	d) Testosterone	
34. Hypersecretion can be defined as;		Answer
a) Too much of a hormone is produced	b) Not enough of a hormone is produced	
c) No hormones are produced	d) A balance of hormones are produced	
35. Which stage of the menstrual cycle does ovulation occur?		Answer
a) Menstrual cycle	b) Secretory phase	
c) Menopause	d) Proliferative phase	
36. Which one of the following is not a function of the cerebrum?		Answer
a) Controls thought and memory	b) Controls feelings of pain	
c) Controls muscle tone and posture	d) Controls conscious movement	
37. What is the largest part of the brain?		Answer
a) The cerebellum	b) The hypothalamus	
c) The brain stem	d) The cerebrum	
38. Which system of the body helps the nervous system to maintain homeostasis?		Answer
a) Respiratory system	b) Endocrine system	
c) Muscular system	d) Circulatory system	
39. The coccygeal plexus is located;		Answer
a) Front of the pelvic cavity	b) Right side of the pelvic cavity	
c) Left side of the pelvic cavity	d) Back of the pelvic cavity	
40. The peripheral nervous system contains;		Answer
a) Brain	b) Spinal cord	
c) Autonomic nervous system	d) Muscle fibres	

41. What is the first part of the birth canal?		Answer
a) Uterus	b) Cervix	
c) Vagina	d) Fallopian tubes	
42. What is the function of the pelvic girdle?		Answer
a) Maintains shape	b) Heat	
c) Protection	d) Protects the abdominal muscles	
43. Which one of the following is not a function of the scrotum?		Answer
a) To store sperm	b) To support the testes	
c) To protect the testes	d) To keep the testes at a lower temperature than the rest of the body	
44. The female sex cells are called;		Answer
a) Ova	b) Sperm	
c) Glans	d) Ovaries	
45. Peptones are broken down into;		Answer
a) Proteins	b) Peptidase	
c) Polypeptides	d) Amino acids	
46. What organ secretes intestinal juices?		Answer
a) Small intestine	b) Liver	
c) Gall bladder	d) Pancreas	
47. Which one of the following is not stored by the liver?		Answer
a) Iron	b) Vitamin E	
c) Glycogen	d) Vitamin B6	
48. What is the chief muscle of respiration?		Answer
a) Intercostal muscles	b) Rectus abdominis	
c) Transverse abdominis	d) Diaphragm	
49. What is the trachea lined with?		
a) Mucus membrane	b) Ciliated epithelium	
c) Serous membrane	d) Squamous epithelial cells	
50. What do bronchioles arise from?		
a) Trachea	b) Alveoli	
c) Terminal bronchioles	d) Bronchi	

Paper 6

1. What type of tissue is adipose tissue?		Answer
a) Nervous tissue	b) Permeable tissue	
c) Elastic tissue	d) Fatty tissue	
2. An area of cytoplasm which contains the centrioles is called?		Answer
a) Chromatid	b) Centromere	
c) Chromosome	d) Centrosome	
3. The transport of substances in a cell is helped by;		Answer
a) Ribosomes	b) Mitochondria	
c) Endoplasmic Reticulum	d) Lysosomes	
4. In which phase of mitosis does the nucleolus disappear?		Answer
a) Interphase	b) Telophase	
c) Prophase	d) Anaphase	
5. Leukonychia describes;		Answer
a) Cracking of the skin around the nail plate	b) White spots on the nail	
c) Flaking nails	d) Forward growth of the cuticle	
6. Which one of the following cannot be absorbed by the skin?		Answer
a) Drugs	b) Water	
c) Almond oil	d) Essential oils	
7. Which one of the following is the resting stage of hair growth?		Answer
a) Anagen	b) Interphase	
c) Catagen	d) Telogen	
8. What do Eccrine glands excrete?		Answer
a) Milky fluid	b) Oil	
c) Sebum	d) Watery sweat	
9. What type of skin disorder is a port wine stain?		Answer
a) Bacterial	b) Fungal	
c) Viral	d) Pigmentation	
10. Desquamation occurs on which layer of the skin?		Answer
a) Stratum spinosum	b) Stratum lucidum	
c) Granular layer	d) Stratum corneum	
11. Which bone joins the foot to the leg?		Answer
a) Navicular	b) Cuboid	
c) Cuneiform	d) Talus	

Anatomy & Physiology Student Workbook

12. What is the structure of slightly moveable joints?		Answer
a) Protective pads of fibrocartilage between the bones	b) Muscular tissue between the bones	
c) Fibrous tissue between the ends of the bones	d) A pad of fibrocartilage between the ends of bones	
13. A bone disease;		Answer
a) Osteoporosis	b) Rheumatoid arthritis	
c) Fracture	d) Slipped disc	
14. Which part of the vertebral column carries the ribs?		Answer
a) Thoracic	b) Lumbar	
c) Cervical	d) Coccygeal	
15. How many bones do the cervical vertebrae contain;		Answer
a) 12	b) 5	
c) 4	d) 7	
16. Where is the risorius positioned?		Answer
a) Around the eye	b) From the masseter to the corner of the mouth	
c) Behind the cheek bone	d) Upper eyelid	
17. What is the deepest muscle of the abdomen?		Answer
a) Transverse abdominis	b) Rectus abdominis	
c) Internal oblique	d) External oblique	
18. Which one of the following is not a function of muscle?		Answer
a) Produce movement	b) Maintain posture	
c) Production of heat	d) Protects organs	
19. What muscle draws the scapula forward?		Answer
a) Serratus anterior	b) Middle deltoid	
c) Internal oblique	d) Posterior deltoid	
20. The function of monocytes is to;		Answer
a) To produce antibodies	b) Transport oxygen as oxyhaemoglobin around the body	
c) Defend the system against micro-organisms	d) Eat bacteria and other micro-organisms	
21. Which layer of the heart contains cardiac muscle?		Answer
a) Pericardium	b) Septum	
c) Myocardium	d) Endocardium	

22. What is the rhesus factor?		Answer
a) An antigen found in white blood cells	b) An antigen found in red blood cells of most people	
c) An antigen found in white blood cells of all animals	d) An antigen found on the surface of red blood cells in most people and animals	
23. Diastolic relates to;		Answer
a) When the heart is contracting	b) When the heart is in a period of relaxation	
c) When the heart is pumping blood around the body	d) High blood pressure	
24. Where is the right lymphatic duct positioned?		Answer
a) Chest	b) Leg	
c) Arm	d) Neck	
25. The submandibular nodes are located;		Answer
a) Face	b) Arms	
c) Legs	d) Chest	
26. The outer layer of lymphatic vessels consist of;		Answer
a) Muscular tissue	b) Elastic tissue	
c) Fibrous tissue	d) Endothelial cells	
27. What is the function of calcitonin?		Answer
a) Helps glucose enter cells	b) Controls body rhythms	
c) Controls calcium levels in the blood	d) Sexual development	
28. An endocrine gland;		Answer
a) Is a chemical messenger	b) A ductless gland which produces hormones	
c) A hormone	d) A ductless gland	
29. What is the function of melanocyte stimulating hormone?		Answer
a) Stimulates the release of melanin	b) Controls the activity of the thyroid gland	
c) Controls sexual development	d) Regulates salts in the body	
30. What hormone is not produced by the anterior lobe of the pituitary gland?		Answer
a) TSH	b) ACTH	
c) Calcitonin	d) Gonadotrophins	
31. Which glands are situated on top of each kidney?		Answer
a) Thyroid glands	b) Pituitary glands	
c) Parathyroids	d) Adrenal glands	

32. Which part of the brain helps with the regulation of metabolism?		Answer
a) Hypothalamus	b) Cerebrum	
c) Midbrain	d) Cerebellum	
33. What disease of the nervous system causes the nerve cells in the brain and spinal cord to lose communication with each other?		Answer
a) Hodgkin's Disease	b) Neuritis	
c) Parkinson's Disease	d) Multiple Sclerosis	
34. The function of the axon is to;		Answer
a) Carry nerve impulses away from the cell body	b) Carry cell bodies away from the nerve impulses	
c) Carry nerve impulses to the cell body	d) Carry nerve impulses away from the neuron	
35. Where is the sciatic nerve located?		Answer
a) Coccygeal plexus	b) Lumbar plexus	
c) Sacral plexus	d) Thoracic plexus	
36. How many pairs of spinal nerves does the spinal cord have?		Answer
a) 13	b) 12	
c) 31	d) 21	
37. What is a zygote?		Answer
a) A ball of cells	b) A fluid filled sac	
c) Tail of the sperm	d) First single cell of an individual	
38. What is the cause of virilism in females?		Answer
a) Hypersecretion of luteinising hormone	b) Hypersecretion of testosterone	
c) Hyposecretion of female sex hormones	d) Hyposecretion of testosterone	
39. What part of the male reproductive system produces testosterone?		Answer
a) Epididymis	b) Testes	
c) Prostate gland	d) Urethra	
40. What do graafian follicles contain?		Answer
a) The ovum	b) Tissue and fluid	
c) Vulva and fluid	d) Nerve endings	
41. Which one of the following is a function of the penis?		Answer
a) Produce testosterone	b) Organ of reproduction	
c) To protect the testes	d) Storage	
42. An obstruction in a bile duct causes;		Answer
a) Hernia	b) Cirrhosis	
c) Gall stones	d) Jaundice	

43. What is the principal organ of digestion?		Answer
a) Stomach	b) Oesophagus	
c) Small intestine	d) Large intestine	
44. Pancreatic juice contains which one of the following enzymes?		Answer
a) Lipase	b) Fibrinogen	
c) Albumin	d) Globulin	
45. What is the function of the oesophagus?		Answer
a) To push the ball of food into the back of the mouth	b) To produce mucus to lubricate food	
c) To eliminate nutrients from digestive waste	d) To convey chewed food downwards towards the stomach	
46. What makes up the small intestine?		Answer
a) Oesophagus and duodenum	b) Duodenum, jejunum and oesophagus	
c) Duodenum, hilium and ileum	d) Duodenum, jejunum and ileum	
47. What is the structure of the trachea?		Answer
a) Incomplete rings of hyaline cartilage and voluntary muscle	b) Connective tissue	
c) Muscular and connective tissue	d) Rings of hyaline cartilage and involuntary muscle	
48. Where is the larynx positioned?		
a) Between the pharynx and the trachea	b) Between the trachea and oesophagus	
c) At the back of the trachea	d) Between the tongue and pharynx	
49. What are the lungs surrounded by?		
a) Goblet cells	b) A membrane called the pleura	
c) Ciliated epithelium	d) Serous epithelium	
50. Inflammation of the bronchial tubes is known as;		
a) Emphysema	b) Bronchitis	
c) Pleurisy	d) Pneumonia	

Paper 7

1. What is the function of areolar tissue?		Answer
a) Protection and elasticity	b) To reduce heat loss	
c) To connect and support	d) To provide attachment	
2. The study of cells and tissue is called;		Answer
a) Histology	b) Physiology	
c) Homeostasis	d) Meiosis	
3. What part of the cell stores and transports the protein out of the cell?		Answer
a) Ribosomes	b) Mitochondria	
c) Golgi apparatus	d) Nucleus	
4. Which one of the following is a function of the nucleus?		Answer
a) To secrete waste materials and transport them out of the cell membrane	b) To control the cell's functions	
c) To form the circulation of a cell	d) Cell reproduction	
5. Where are goblet cells found?		Answer
a) Columnar epithelium	b) Squamous epithelium	
c) Compound epithelium	d) Cuboidal epithelium	
6. Metabolism describes;		Answer
a) The physiological processes of the cell	b) The physiological processes of the body	
c) The physiological processes of the tissues	d) The psychological processes of the body	
7. When does the inner root sheath stop growing?		Answer
a) When it is level with the dermal papilla	b) When it is level with the sebaceous gland	
c) When it is level with the matrix	d) When it is level with the outer root sheath	
8. The top layer of the epidermis is known as;		Answer
a) Stratum lucidum	b) Stratum corneum	
c) Stratum spinosum	d) Stratum germinativum	
9. How would you recognize paronychia?		Answer
a) Swollen, inflamed red skin around the nail, pus may be present	b) Small patches of red skin at the base of the nail, with silvery scales	
c) Large areas of white or yellow patches on the nail	d) Grooves in the nail plate running from the base of the nail to the free edge	

Anatomy & Physiology Student Workbook

10. Hyperaemia can be defined as;		Answer
a) A reduction in the blood's ability to carry oxygen	b) An increase of blood flow in the body causing the skin to become hot and flush	
c) When the body becomes cold, body hair stands on end, raising the body temperature	d) When sweat and sebum form a protective barrier on the skin	
11. Liver spots are also known as;		Answer
a) Vitiligo	b) Lentigo	
c) Ephelides	d) Naevae	
12. Superficial describes;		Answer
a) Nearer to the midline of the body	b) The outer surface of the body	
c) Nearer to the surface	d) Towards the higher part	
13. The metacarpals are known as;		Answer
a) Finger bones	b) Toe bones	
c) Palm bones	d) Ankle bones	
14. Which bone is positioned on the inside of each arm towards the thumb?		Answer
a) Radius	b) Humerus	
c) Capitate	d) Ulna	
15. Fixed vertebrae are;		Answer
a) Cervical	b) Sacral and coccygeal	
c) Lumbar	d) Thoracic	
16. What muscle helps with chewing?		Answer
a) Buccinator	b) Masseter	
c) Orbicularis oculi	d) Depressor anguli oris	
17. Which one of the following is not a cause of a strain?		Answer
a) Over use	b) Over exertion	
c) Over stretching	d) Over heating	
18. Smooth muscle is also known as;		Answer
a) Skeletal muscle	b) Involuntary muscle	
c) Voluntary muscle	d) Cardiac muscle	
19. What is the action of the gastrocnemius?		Answer
a) Flexes toes	b) Extends toes	
c) Extends foot	d) Plantarflexes foot	

20. Fibromyalgia affects what part of the body?		Answer
a) Lower back	b) Hands	
c) Back, neck and shoulders	d) Face	
21. Patients with which blood type can receive any blood group?		Answer
a) Type O	b) Type A	
c) Type AB	d) Type B	
22. Hypotension is also known as;		Answer
a) Low blood pressure	b) High blood pressure	
c) Blood clotting	d) Anaemia	
23. What are the 2 categories of leucocytes?		Answer
a) Monocytes and granulocytes	b) Lymphocytes and thrombocytes	
c) Granulocytes and agranulocytes	d) Granulocytes and phagocytes	
24. What do most venules unite to form?		Answer
a) Arteries	b) Ventricles	
c) Capillaries	d) Veins	
25. Trabecula are;		Answer
a) Inward strands of elastic tissue	b) Inward strands of fibrous tissue	
c) Inward strands of lymphatic tissue	d) Inward strands of muscular tissue	
26. The occipital nodes are located;		Answer
a) On the face	b) At the back of the skull	
c) Armpits	d) Elbows	
27. An afferent vessel carries lymph;		Answer
a) Around the body	b) To the lymph ducts	
c) To the lymph nodes	d) To lymph capillaries	
28. Which of the following is a function of interstitial cell stimulating hormone?		Answer
a) Maintains BMR	b) Regulates water absorption in kidneys	
c) Stimulate testosterone production in males	d) Regulates salts in the body	
29. Where are T Cells found?		Answer
a) Pituitary gland	b) Thyroid gland	
c) Thymus	d) Adrenal medulla	
30. Hyposecretion of parathormone causes;		Answer
a) Cushing's syndrome	b) Tetany	
c) Low blood sugar levels	d) Diabetes insipidus	

31. What hormone stimulates testosterone production in men?		Answer
a) Interstitial cell stimulating hormone	b) Follicle stimulating hormone	
c) Lactogenic hormone	d) Adrenocorticotrophin	
32. Which of the following is not a function of the myelin sheath?		Answer
a) Pass on the nerve impulse to the dendrites	b) Insulates the axon	
c) Accelerates the conduction of nerves	d) Protects the axon from pressure	
33. Ganglia is another term for;		Answer
a) A collection of nerve endings	b) Nerve tissue	
c) A collection of neurones	d) A collection of reflexes	
34. Cerebrospinal fluid;		Answer
a) Is a clear liquid inside and around the brain	b) Is a yellow fluid situated in the lining of the brain	
c) Is a double layer of tough fibrous membrane	d) Is a thin vascular membrane	
35. Which part of the meninges supplies blood to the brain and spinal cord?		Answer
a) Dura mater	b) Outer membrane	
c) Pia mater	d) Arachnoid mater	
36. What is the uterus lined with?		Answer
a) Endometrium	b) Fibrous tissue	
c) Graafian follicle	d) Placenta	
37. The prepuce is another term for;		Answer
a) Foreskin	b) Tip of the penis	
c) Erectile tissue	d) Sperm	
38. What is the function of the labia majora?		Answer
a) To protect the other external female reproductive organs	b) To protect the symphysis pubis	
c) To protect the clitoris	d) To protect the labia minora	
39. Where do immature sperm cells develop?		Answer
a) Epididymis	b) Vas deferens	
c) Scrotum	d) Testes	
40. Where are taste buds located?		Answer
a) On the tongue	b) In saliva	
c) Oesophagus	d) Lips	

41. Food leaves the stomach through the;		Answer
a) Pyloric sphincter	b) Cardiac sphincter	
c) Oesophagus	d) Large intestine	
42. What enzyme splits proteins into peptones?		Answer
a) Peptidase	b) Polypeptides	
c) Trypsin	d) Pepsin	
43. What is the function of the small intestine?		Answer
a) To absorb nutrients into the bloodstream	b) To emulsify fats and carbohydrates	
c) To remove waste	d) To begin the production of intestinal juices	
44. What is the structure of the diaphragm?		Answer
a) Flat shaped muscle with ligaments and tendons	b) A large dome shaped sheet of muscle	
c) A large dome shaped muscle with a sheet of tendon with muscle fibres	d) U shaped muscle with muscle & nerve fibres	
45. Which part of the respiratory system takes air to the alveoli of the lungs?		Answer
a) Pleura	b) Bronchioles	
c) Bronchi	d) Capillaries	
46. What are the lungs surrounded by?		Answer
a) Goblet cells	b) A membrane called the pleura	
c) Ciliated epithelium	d) Serous epithelium	
47. What is the structure of the bladder?		Answer
a) A funnel shaped organ	b) A funnel shaped cavity	
c) A bean shaped organ	d) A hollow sac like organ	
48. What acts as the first step in the filtration of blood to form urine?		Answer
a) Bowman's capsule	b) Glomerulus	
c) Nephron	d) Loop of henle	
49. The cortex is located;		Answer
a) On the inside of the kidney	b) Pelvis	
c) On the outside of the kidney	d) Gall bladder	
50. What is the function of the Bowman's Capsule?		Answer
a) Absorption of waste products	b) Acts as a passageway for urine through the kidneys	
c) Acts as the first step for filtering blood in the kidneys	d) To carry waste products from the glomerulus to the loop of henle	

Paper 8

1. Which type of tissue protects and supports?		Answer
a) Connective	b) Muscular	
c) Nervous	d) Epithelium	
2. Anabolism describes;		Answer
a) The minimum energy required to keep the body going	b) The process of engulfing foreign particles	
c) The process of building up complex substances from simple molecules	d) The process of storing energy	
3. At the anaphase of mitosis the;		Answer
a) The centrioles separate and form spindle fibres	b) Identical pairs of chromosomes move to one end of the cell and the other pairs move to the other end	
c) Centrosome divides into 2 centrioles	d) Cell is resting	
4. What is the function of ribosomes?		Answer
a) To supply the cell with energy	b) To allow movement of substances throughout the cell	
c) To produce protein	d) Control the cell	
5. What is the function of white fibrous tissue?		Answer
a) Insulatory	b) Stretching	
c) Supports organs	d) Protecting and supporting surrounding structures	
6. What layer of the hair contains melanin?		Answer
a) Cuticle	b) Medulla	
c) Vellus	d) Cortex	
7. Tinea pedis is commonly referred to as;		Answer
a) Ringworm	b) Athlete's foot	
c) Cold sore	d) Shingles	
8. Which one of the following nail diseases describes the thickening of the nail plate?		Answer
a) Onychocryptosis	b) Onychauxis	
c) Pterygium	d) Onychophagy	
9. When the skin becomes too warm it automatically cools itself down. What is this process called?		Answer
a) Vasodilation	b) Heat regulation	
c) Vasoconstriction	d) Absorption	

10. The clear layer of the epidermis;		Answer
a) Stratum germinativum	b) Stratum lucidum	
c) Stratum spinosum	d) Stratum corneum	
11. The anatomical term that describes being further from the surface is;		Answer
a) Medial	b) Superficial	
c) Proximal	d) Deep	
12. What are cartilage forming cells called?		Answer
a) Chondrocytes	b) Osteoclasts	
c) Erythrocytes	d) Thrombocytes	
13. What type of joint allows movement in 2 directions?		Answer
a) Condyloid	b) Pivot	
c) Fibrous	d) Hinge	
14. Which one of the following is not a wrist bone?		Answer
a) Trapezium	b) Capitate	
c) Lunate	d) Medial	
15. Which one of the following is a type of irregular bone?		Answer
a) Sphenoid	b) Lacrimal	
c) Metacarpals	d) Scapula	
16. What is the action of the extensor pollicus longus?		Answer
a) Extends wrist	b) Flexes wrist	
c) Extends thumb	d) Extends little finger	
17. Which one of the following is not an action of the latissimus dorsi?		Answer
a) Draws arm backwards	b) Adducts the arm	
c) Rotates the arm medially	d) Abducts the arm	
18. Which muscle pulls the lower lip out?		Answer
a) Depressor anguli oris	b) Masseter	
c) Medial pterygoid	d) Mentalis	
18. Adduction describes;		Answer
a) Moving a limb away from the midline	b) Moving a limb towards the midline	
c) Turning a limb to face upwards	d) Turning a limb towards the centre	
19. Muscle that relaxes to allow the prime mover to contract;		Answer
a) The insertion	b) The antagonist	
c) The muscle belly	d) The agonist	

20. The blood is pushed from the right atrium into the right ventricle through;		Answer
a) Micuspid valve	b) Tricuspid valve	
c) Septum valve	d) Bicuspid valve	
21. Which one of the following is one of the main veins of the legs?		Answer
a) Brachial	b) Cephalic	
c) Axillary	d) Anterior tibial	
22. Deoxygenated blood travels from the upper body into the right atrium via;		Answer
a) Pulmonary veins	b) Superior vena cava	
c) Pulmonary artery	d) Inferior vena cava	
23. Enzymes are described as;		Answer
a) Hormones	b) Chemical substances in the body	
c) Oxygen and carbon dioxide	d) Chemical messengers in the blood	
24. Which plasma protein changes fibrinogen into fibrin?		Answer
a) Albumin	b) Thrombin	
c) Adrenaline	d) Thromboplastin	
25. What is lymphadenitis?		Answer
a) Inflammation of lymphatic capillaries	b) Inflammation of lymphatic vessels	
c) Inflammation of lymphatic tissue	d) Inflammation of lymph nodes	
26. How many layers do lymphatic vessels have?		Answer
a) 3	b) 2	
c) 4	d) 1	
27. The supratrochlear nodes are located;		Answer
a) Behind the ears	b) Armpits	
c) Behind the knees	d) Elbows	
28. What is the function of antidiuretic hormone?		Answer
a) Stimulates basic metabolic rate	b) Increases water reabsorption in kidneys	
c) Maintains calcium levels in bones	d) Contracts the uterus during labour	
29. Hyposecretion of insulin causes;		Answer
a) Hypoglycaemia	b) Diabetes insipidus	
c) Sweating	d) Diabetes mellitus	
30. Which one of the following is a function of the hormones produced by the thyroid glands?		Answer
a) Regulates metabolism	b) Regulates blood sugar levels	
c) Produces vitamin D	d) Regulates salt levels	

31. Which one of the following is not an effect of Cushing's syndrome?		Answer
a) Weight gain	b) Low blood pressure	
c) Muscle weakness	d) Mental illness	
32. The start of menstruation is known as;		Answer
a) Menopause	b) Menarche	
c) Proliferative	d) Menstrual cycle	
33. Motor nerves are also known as;		Answer
a) Afferent nerves	b) Grey matter	
c) Sensory nerves	d) Efferent nerves	
34. What muscle type does the autonomic nervous system control?		Answer
a) Striated and involuntary	b) Cardiac and skeletal	
c) Skeletal and smooth	d) Smooth and cardiac	
35. Which one of the following is not a function of the hypothalamus?		Answer
a) Regulation of the pituitary gland	b) Controls body temperature	
c) Regulation of hunger and thirst	d) Secretion of melatonin	
36. Which one of the following is not a function of the sympathetic nervous system?		Answer
a) Slows heart rate	b) Releases noradrenaline preparing the body for fight or flight	
c) Increases inspiration	d) Increases blood supply to the heart	
37. Which part of the body do the thoracic nerves supply?		Answer
a) Thighs	b) Chest	
c) Fingertips	d) Neck	
38. What is the function of the mons pubis?		Answer
a) To protect the entrance to the vagina	b) Form a hood to protect the clitoris	
c) To form part of the birth canal	d) To protect the symphysis pubis	
39. Which one of the following is contained within the scrotum?		Answer
a) Testes	b) Erectile tissue	
c) Seminal fluid	d) Prostate	
40. The womb is also called;		Answer
a) Follicle	b) Cervix	
c) Uterus	d) Vulva	

Anatomy & Physiology Student Workbook

41. What part of the male reproductive system leads from the epididymis to the urethra?		Answer
a) Prostate gland	b) Vas deferens	
c) Ureter	d) Erectile tissue	
42. Which one of the following is not a function of the liver?		Answer
a) Secretion of bile	b) Removes toxins	
c) Production of heat	d) Production of enzymes to break down food	
43. Motor nerves are also known as;		Answer
a) Afferent nerves	b) Grey matter	
c) Sensory nerves	d) Efferent nerves	
44. A disaccharide is a type of;		Answer
a) Pancreatic juice	b) Fat	
c) Protein	d) Carbohydrate	
45. What is the function of the cardiac sphincter?		Answer
a) To prevent choking	b) To control the movement of food into the stomach	
c) To carry food to the small intestine	d) To carry food to the large intestine	
46. What is the function of salivary amylase?		Answer
a) Begins the digestion of starch	b) Converts milk into curds	
c) Changes fats into fatty acids	d) Begins the digestion of proteins	
47. External respiration is another term for;		Answer
a) Inhalation	b) Exhalation	
c) Breathing	d) Exchange of gases	
48. What is the structure of the alveoli?		Answer
a) A single layer of squamous epithelial cells	b) A thick layer of serous membrane	
c) A thick layer of squamous epithelial cells lined with ciliated membrane	d) A thin layer of ciliated epithelial cells	
49. BCG vaccines are used to prevent which disease?		Answer
a) Pneumonia	b) Tuberculosis	
c) Rhinitis	d) Emphysema	
50. What part of the respiratory system carries air to the lungs from the trachea?		Answer
a) Larynx	b) Oesophagus	
c) Bronchi	d) Bronchioles	

Mock Exam Paper Answers

Paper 1

1	A	11	B	21	B	31	A	41	A
2	A	12	D	22	A	32	B	42	C
3	B	13	D	23	C	33	C	43	B
4	C	14	C	24	B	34	D	44	B
5	A	15	D	25	D	35	B	45	C
6	B	16	B	26	A	36	B	46	A
7	D	17	C	27	A	37	C	47	D
8	C	18	B	28	C	38	B	48	B
9	A	19	D	29	B	39	D	49	C
10	A	20	B	30	D	40	B	50	D

Paper 2

1	C	11	C	21	C	31	D	41	B
2	D	12	A	22	D	32	C	42	A
3	D	13	A	23	C	33	A	43	D
4	B	14	C	24	A	34	A	44	A
5	B	15	D	25	C	35	A	45	C
6	C	16	B	26	A	36	C	46	B
7	A	17	C	27	A	37	C	47	A
8	C	18	A	28	A	38	D	48	A
9	D	19	A	29	B	39	A	49	A
10	D	20	B	30	C	40	D	50	B

Paper 3

1	C	11	B	21	B	31	A	41	C
2	B	12	A	22	A	32	B	42	D
3	D	13	C	23	D	33	D	43	B
4	B	14	C	24	B	34	C	44	D
5	A	15	B	25	A	35	B	45	A
6	D	16	D	26	A	36	C	46	C
7	A	17	D	27	B	37	B	47	C
8	B	18	C	28	B	38	B	48	C
9	C	19	B	29	B	39	A	49	A
10	C	20	B	30	B	40	C	50	D

Anatomy & Physiology Student Workbook

Paper 4

1	D	11	B	21	A	31	D	41	D
2	C	12	D	22	A	32	B	42	D
3	A	13	D	23	B	33	A	43	C
4	C	14	A	24	A	34	B	44	C
5	D	15	A	25	D	35	B	45	B
6	C	16	B	26	B	36	C	46	A
7	D	17	A	27	C	37	A	47	A
8	A	18	D	28	B	38	C	48	C
9	A	19	D	29	B	39	D	49	B
10	C	20	C	30	D	40	B	50	B

Paper 5

1	A	11	B	21	C	31	C	41	B
2	D	12	C	22	A	32	B	42	C
3	A	13	D	23	D	33	B	43	A
4	C	14	C	24	D	34	A	44	A
5	D	15	B	25	B	35	D	45	C
6	A	16	A	26	A	36	C	46	A
7	B	17	B	27	A	37	D	47	D
8	A	18	A	28	D	38	B	48	D
9	C	19	A	29	C	39	D	49	B
10	B	20	A	30	C	40	C	50	D

Paper 6

1	D	11	D	21	C	31	D	41	B
2	D	12	A	22	D	32	A	42	D
3	C	13	A	23	B	33	D	43	A
4	C	14	A	24	D	34	A	44	A
5	B	15	D	25	A	35	C	45	D
6	B	16	B	26	C	36	C	46	D
7	D	17	A	27	C	37	D	47	D
8	D	18	D	28	B	38	B	48	A
9	D	19	A	29	A	39	B	49	B
10	D	20	D	30	C	40	A	50	B

Paper 7

1	C	11	B	21	C	31	A	41	A
2	A	12	C	22	A	32	A	42	D
3	C	13	C	23	C	33	C	43	A
4	B	14	A	24	D	34	A	44	C
5	A	15	B	25	B	35	C	45	B
6	B	16	A	26	B	36	A	46	B
7	B	17	D	27	C	37	A	47	D
8	B	18	B	28	C	38	A	48	A
9	A	19	D	29	C	39	A	49	C
10	B	20	C	30	B	40	A	50	C

Paper 8

1	A	11	D	21	D	31	B	41	B
2	C	12	A	22	B	32	B	42	D
3	B	13	A	23	B	33	D	43	D
4	C	14	D	24	B	34	D	44	D
5	D	15	A	25	D	35	D	45	B
6	D	16	C	26	A	36	A	46	A
7	B	17	D	27	D	37	B	47	C
8	B	18	D	28	B	38	D	48	A
9	A	19	B	29	D	39	A	49	B
10	B	20	B	30	A	40	C	50	C

Anatomy & Physiology Student Workbook

Printed in Great Britain
by Amazon